# WHEN SCIENCE SHEDS LIGHT ON HISTORY

UNIVERSITY PRESS OF FLORIDA

Florida A&M University, Tallahassee
Florida Atlantic University, Boca Raton
Florida Gulf Coast University, Ft. Myers
Florida International University, Miami
Florida State University, Tallahassee
New College of Florida, Sarasota
University of Central Florida, Orlando
University of Florida, Gainesville
University of North Florida, Jacksonville
University of South Florida, Tampa
University of West Florida, Pensacola

BY THE SAME AUTHOR

*Zombis: Enquête sur les morts-vivants*, Paris, Tallandier, 2015

*Quand la science explore l'histoire*, in collaboration with David Alliot, Paris, Tallandier, 2014.

(ed.) *Seine de crime*. Paris, Le Rocher, 2014.

(ed.) *Actes du 4ᵉ colloque international de pathographie* (Saint-Jean-de-Côle, May 2011), in collaboration with D. Gourevitch, Paris, De Boccard, *Pathographie* 9, 2013.

*Henri IV, l'énigme du roi sans tête*, in collaboration with S. Gabet, Paris, Vuibert, 2013.

*Paris au scalpel: Itinéraires secrets d'un médecin légiste*, Paris, Le Rocher, 2012.

*Autopsie de l'art premier*, Paris, Le Rocher, 2012.

*Les secrets des grands crimes de l'histoire*, Paris, Vuibert, 2012.

(ed.) *Le miroir du temps: Les momies de Randazzo (XVIIᵉ–XIXᵉ siècle)*, in collaboration with L. Lo Gerfo, Paris, De Boccard, *Pathographie* 7, 2011.

(ed.) *Le roman des morts secrètes de l'histoire*, Paris, Le Rocher, 2011.

(ed.) *Actes du 3ᵉ colloque international de pathographie* (Bourges, April 2009), Paris, De Boccard, *Pathographie* 6, 2011.

(ed.) *Actes du 2ᵉ colloque international de pathographie* (Loches, April 2007), Paris, De Boccard, *Pathographie* 4, 2009.

*Male mort: Morts violentes dans l'Antiquité*, Paris, Fayard, 2009.

*Les jeunes filles et la mort: Catalogue de l'exposition*, Bourges, Les 1000 univers, 2009.

*Maladies humaines, thérapies divines: Analyse épigraphique et paléopathologique de textes de guérison grecs*, in collaboration with C. Prêtre, Lille, PUS, 2009.

(ed.) *Ostéo-archéologie et techniques médico-légales*, Paris, De Boccard, *Pathographie* 2, 2008.

*Les monstres humains dans l'Antiquité: Analyse paléopathologique*, Paris, Fayard, 2008.

(ed.) *Actes du 1ᵉʳ colloque international de pathographie* (Loches, April 2005), Paris, De Boccard, *Pathographie* 1, 2007.

*Médecin des morts: Récits de paléopathologie*, Paris, Fayard, 2006; Pluriel, 2014.

# WHEN SCIENCE
# SHEDS LIGHT ON HISTORY

## FORENSIC SCIENCE AND ANTHROPOLOGY

## PHILIPPE CHARLIER

with David Alliot

Translated by Isabelle Ruben

University Press of Florida

Gainesville · Tallahassee · Tampa · Boca Raton

Pensacola · Orlando · Miami · Jacksonville · Ft. Myers · Sarasota

# CONTENTS

## PART IV. RENAISSANCE TO MODERN TIMES

# AUTHOR'S PREFACE TO THE ENGLISH EDITION

The various branches of the fundamental and life sciences should not be so distinctly divided. The benefits of a multidisciplinary approach have been demonstrated, and we hope that this book will be no exception to the rule. In France, over the last ten years or so, our team has been keen to ensure interaction between forensic science and osteoarchaeology. The patients—and we can rightly call them patients because it is doctors who examine these human remains, be they ancient or modern, complete or incomplete, anonymous or clearly identified—are countless (in the tens of thousands). First, there is the impressive number of skeletons, mummies, and anatomical parts that have no biographical data: these are the anonymous ones, bodies without names, who make history. These bodies—from Roman and medieval necropolises, ossuaries of lepers, communal burial pits from the First World War, collective graves from the Neolithic and so on—form the major part of our work. Then there are clearly identified remains for which we have biographical information (at least a name, the age at death, a portrait, the causes or circumstances of death, or an epitaph; in other words, at least some details that mean we are not working blind): these are the identified ones, the named bodies, who make history; this branch of the discipline is known as pathography.

The whole point of this "mixing of types," far from being academic diversification, is to improve techniques for the identification of individuals and retrospective diagnosis, for the benefit of both forensic science (and therefore of justice) and history. A few examples (which are explored in this book) of procedures that have been improved thanks to the examination in our laboratories of historical figures include facial reconstructions, based on the contours of the cranium or on death masks of patients such as Henri IV and Robespierre; the levels of gold or mercury in hair, for

Diane de Poitiers and Agnès Sorel; protocols for the analysis of carbonized remains, for the "remains of Joan of Arc"; the distinction between pre- and post-mortem tattooing for Maori heads from New Zealand, etc.

The dead are absolutely everywhere. The whole world is peopled by cadavers, and we spend our time walking over them. They are "the most numerous," to use an ancient Greek expression. So many patients to examine, so many dead to give a voice to, to save from oblivion. So many dead who are useful to the living, to make us remember. Amabu Hampate Ba's phrase is well known: "When an old man dies, a library burns"; the same can be said of ancient remains, because every skeleton that turns to dust is a sum of knowledge about the past that disappears forever.

# PREFACE

The dead are useful to the living. One must speak with the ancestors, or rather, make them speak, to discover the past. Even using just a bone or a fragment of bone. This is the profession of the forensic scientist. For Justice, the forensic scientist creates scenarios based on successive snapshots built up from his studies of the dead body. But some bodies, or parts of bodies, belong to history. Through a saga stretching from Prehistory to Robespierre via Joan of Arc and Henri IV, Philippe Charlier revisits the history of our world using a new scientific light to gain a better understanding of the lives of our ancestors and the societies in which they lived. This book is a scientific and cultural journey through time and space that bears witness to great curiosity. Like a navigator charting his course, Philippe Charlier is there where no one expects him, in other words, somewhere else. He shows up at Buthiers-Boulancourt, in Egypt, Greece, Rome, Romania, Bourges. . . . Curiosity is a unique quality. As Erik Orsenna has written: "Inquisitive people take care of the world."

On this voyage, which includes about forty ports of call described in this work in a sometimes-playful manner, Philippe Charlier is not alone. His work is the fruit of numerous meetings and exchanges in a multidisciplinary setting. Intended mainly for the general public, this book is based on scientific work, cited in the references, with a dynamic interaction between osteoarchaeology and forensic anthropology. Charlier's study program, which gained him the qualification to direct research in medical biology in 2013, after the presentation of his PhD thesis in 2012, was aimed at developing the use of biomedical and osteoarchaeological techniques in forensic science—principally in anthropology, but also on biological traces and isolated body fragments. The intention was to improve the means of identifying individuals and retrospective diagnoses—the underlying pathological condition and the causes and circumstances of death. Charlier's work centered on improving techniques and the description of new entities in this setting.

These historical, retrospective studies also provide a way of testing methods and scientific protocols that are useful in forensic science. History, the exploration of the past, helps us to catch a glimpse of where we came from and where we are going. This is a forward-looking approach. One must remember that the word "history" comes from the Greek *historia* and means "inquiry." The intellectual approach of the historian is close to that of the forensic scientist, who recreates the story of an individual within his or her peer group and at a specific time.

The problem is that Philippe Charlier has a pool of patients consisting of famous people who have already been monitored by others. In a way, he makes counter-inspections. This often raises passionate debates, which is a good thing. Squalls are part of navigation. Let us remember the excitement triggered by the discovery of arsenic in Napoleon's hair: was it intoxication or artifact? And then the evaluations and counter-evaluations that followed, with scientific debates between toxicologists and respected historians to try to identify the cause of this intoxication: Was it poisoning or not? Such dossiers are politically sensitive, because they can upset national history, collective memory and the reputation of important families. In France, incidentally, the forensic scientist has sometimes been a political doctor: I am thinking of forensic pathologists, notably during the Revolution.

On this matter, the story of Robespierre is still being researched today, through the archives and medical and forensic documents. Who shot Robespierre in the face, and with what firearm? Was it attempted homicide, attempted suicide, or an accident? What was Merda's role? Vergez and Marrigues, who worked for the Convention, were called by the representatives of the people making up the Committee of General Security to bandage the wounds of that "criminal" Robespierre. They produced a forensic report, inaccurate and poorly documented to my mind, at the end of which Robespierre was described as a "monster." The independence of the doctors is debatable. Finally, according to the archive documents, Robespierre was sitting or lying down at the moment when he was shot. Today, it would be simple: we would examine a 3D reconstruction of scanner images! With Philippe Froesh, an expert in facial reconstruction, Philippe Charlier analyzed a scientific reconstruction of Robespierre's face based on molds taken of his face. This has shed new light on the matter, and it merits discussion.

Everything is useful for obtaining direct or indirect information on the history of humans: the body—or what is left of it—of course, biological traces, putrefaction liquid, dental tartar, and so on, but also death masks, portraits, medical records, and ancient writings. To exploit all these types of information, one must leave the laboratory and engage in a multidisciplinary approach to pool the abilities and analyze the information produced by the various specialties. It is a sometimes-difficult, but seductive, course to navigate.

Reading the cases presented in this book confirms that there are three different interwoven and complementary outlooks in the professional trajectory and research of Dr. Philippe Charlier: a historical outlook through the study of human remains and their environment for a better understanding of the past; a scientific outlook through the evaluation of new techniques and methods of analysis; and an ethical and social outlook on the status of the dead body.

A final attribute of Philippe Charlier is that he does not leave one indifferent. The passionate debates in the scientific domain are salutary. Perhaps in the next century a new chapter will have to be added, entitled "The real-false head of Philippe Charlier," discovered . . . in the basement of the Ambroise-Paré hospital.

*Prof. Bernard Proust*
*Neurologist, Professor of Forensic Science at the CHU of Rouen*

*The shortest path to the future is always one that runs through the deepening of the past.*

AIMÉ CÉSAIRE

# FOREWORD

Why, in forensic medicine, work on ancient remains? The choice might seem surprising, but in the absolute, there is nothing that so much resembles a forensic case as an ancient archaeological skeleton. The dizzying decline in hospital autopsies and in donations of bodies to scientific research has forced researchers to turn to other sources to further the state of knowledge. Thus human remains that are found in archaeological excavations offer real cases for study and occasionally for experimentation, which allow certain research laboratories to improve the techniques of retrospective diagnosis (demonstrating a specific pathology, a particular activity, etc.) and of personal identification (confirming or refuting a presumed identification of an individual). For some, this is seen as "economizing" on corpses, for others as respect for the recently deceased, and for yet others as legitimate opportunism, but in all cases the dead prove themselves useful to the living.

This book is also the result of many encounters and countless fruitful exchanges. Scientific research is, and owes it to itself to be, objective; so this research is not the result of solitary work in a laboratory, but of the work of a multidisciplinary team, which implies a sound and necessary dialogue between researchers. Some of the studies documented below brought together as many as thirty researchers, some of whom had never worked in forensic medicine before, but who have since become regular collaborators: philologists who helped us understand the meaning and context of inscriptions better; a "nose" from a perfume house who identified precisely, by their smell, the odoriferous products used in embalming (when a reliquary was opened); textile specialists; mathematicians; and so forth.

Working on human remains (be they ancient or recent) undeniably leads one to question the ethics of research and the legitimacy of this anthropological work. Is everything permissible with a dead body? Is it legitimate to open a tomb out of scientific curiosity? Is it all right to conserve a skeleton in an institute for the potential benefit of future research? The answers to these questions are complex, and only a multidisciplinary consideration can bring out the pertinent points. All the cases presented here were "opportunistic": in other words, they were studied in the context of fortuitous discoveries, or the relocation or restoration of a tomb (in order to respect the last wishes of the deceased or to redress historic defilement), etc.

Throughout this book we have used the term "patient" when we speak of these individuals who have come to us from the past. First, because this word seems natural when discussing humans subjects being examined by doctors, often in a university hospital—but also because the term is itself a token of, and witness to, our respect. Before being reduced to a bare skeleton, or crumbling to dust, these remains were, at one point in their history, alive. We owe them genuine respect.

*Philippe Charlier*

# INTRODUCTION

It is hard to believe how much information a human skeleton or even a single bone can provide. Paleopathology—in other words, the medical study of ancient human remains found in archaeological excavations or in museum collections—is becoming more and more significant a scientific discipline. Together with the history of medicine and diseases, archaeology, and physical anthropology, as well as with history, sociology, and demography, it explores all possible and imaginable avenues of research in order to identify diseases based on more or less complete fragments of skeletons and mummies. Isolated cases are as interesting as vast necropolises, each bringing radically different information, and specifically adapted methods are used in each case. We often forget that we have much to learn from the past.

This discipline leads to a better understanding of the lifestyles of those who preceded us, their dietary habits, their ritual practices, the causes of their deaths, and, as a result, the world of the living is easier to grasp. In fact, there is nothing that so much resembles a forensic case as an archaeological skeleton.

Interaction between forensic medicine and osteoarchaeology is relatively recent (thirty years at the most); the consequences have sometimes been astonishing, but are always founded on scientific publications ensuring visibility and integration in the discipline. Identifying gold in Diane de Poitiers' hair and mercury in that of Agnès Sorel led to the substantial modification of doses of these metals in a forensic context. The cremation process of an ancient Greek soldier or the analysis of a Hindu pyre on the banks of the Ganges leads to a better understanding of the criminal incineration of a present-day victim in a car, and helps with the "demonstration of truth," particularly judicially. Certain entities have even been described (such as deposits of putrefaction fluids or dental tartar), the scientific possibilities of which were first tested on ancient subjects before being confirmed on recent legal cases. Archaeological discoveries allow progress each time, to the benefit of the living, in other words, of the "future dead." Finally, this line of research does not consist only of the study of bodies in the strict sense, but also looks at traces and testimonies such as medical records, death masks, portraits, fingerprints, blood stains—in other words, anything that provides direct or indirect testimony on the health or daily life of a particular individual or past populations, and rituals associated with the struggle against the unknown. The applications of this research are vast, and it is likely that some have not yet seen the light of day.

Most of the cases presented here are anonymous, but are undeniably of interest because the rare pathologies that are involved have allowed scientific protocols to be established, which today help to further criminology. A few of the "patients" are famous, like Richard the Lionheart, Joan of Arc, Agnès Sorel, Diane de Poitiers, Henri IV, Robespierre, etc. The choice of these subjects of study is not insignificant: it is because they allow researchers to test, to improve, and to validate the forensic process of individual identification. At the same time, some historical hypotheses can also be confirmed or invalidated.

The forty or so cases presented in this book, stretching from prehistory to the 19th century, are the result of more than ten years' work. The aim is to show the great variety of the objects and of today's methods of study.

Paleopathology leads to a better understanding of the lives of our ancestors, to more detailed historical data, and finally, to a better understanding of ourselves. Today, more than ever, the living need the dead.

# I

## PREHISTORY

# PLANET OF THE WISE

Tending Disabilities during Prehistory

In our contemporary imagination, prehistoric man is often likened to primitive peoples. Stereotypes such as this appeared in the 19th century, popularized in Rosny Aîné's novels about prehistory, such as *Quest for Fire*. They rely largely on false and preconceived notions that, even today, are widely accepted by the general public. Luckily, modern archaeological discoveries have given us other ideas about our distant ancestors. One of the main pieces of received wisdom that needs demolishing is the perception of disability in prehistory.

During prehistory in Europe and beyond, it seems that healthy individuals took care of the elderly, the malformed, the wounded, and invalids, who, contrary to another widespread cliché, were neither excluded nor rejected from the social group. On the contrary, given the nomadism or semi-nomadism of the time, the movement of invalids would be taken care of by the community. For by keeping the wounded, the invalids, and the malformed alive, the group's capacity for reproduction increased, and its survival was ensured *because of their numbers*: deafness or a missing femur has never prevented procreation. The other way of ensuring the group's survival consisted of keeping the ancients with it—survival *by intelligence*, for the ancients were the repositories of wisdom that was important for the whole group. Individual competition did not exist at the time; only the survival of the group was paramount.

Archaeology provides us with greater insight into this human solidarity. For example, some completely toothless human crania have been found. They belonged to elderly people, and careful examination shows that the tooth loss had completely healed—proof that the loss of the teeth had occurred well before death. But without their teeth, these individuals could not have survived, and would eventually have died of hunger. Their survival can be explained by the preparation of food in the form of mush or gruel by the rest of the community. As for a wounded individual, he was taken care of by the rest of the community while immobile and while the wounds were being stabilized and tended. Cases of serious trauma have been found, such as the Mesolithic woman (9000 BC) discovered in Columnata (Morocco), whose fractured pelvis led to the complete paralysis of both her legs; the medical study of this case shows that she survived long after her accident, which would have been impossible without the solidarity of the clan. The same is true for individuals with genetic anomalies or malformations, which may have been a fairly widespread problem during prehistory, given the relatively restricted and inevitably endogamous human groups, even though such a diagnosis is more difficult to make than the previous ones. When a skeleton is examined, there can be some telltale signs on the bones—these could have produced serious exterior anomalies.

On the other hand, though archaeology has brought to light a reasonable number of cases of care within the clan, there is nothing to exclude the possibility that individuals with genetic anomalies or disabilities were sacrificed. But it was clearly an infrequent eventuality. On this point, let us mention the existence of an archaeological case found in Harsova, Romania, dating to the Neolithic (4000–3000 BC). Remains of two sacrificed children, feet and hands tied, were found in a pit under some dwellings. These two children were malformed or crippled. For the community, it was probably a case of sacrificing two individuals who were incompatible with useful physical activity and at the same time maintaining a religious custom (of human sacrifice for the foundation of a new building).

Generally, looking after "invalids" was accepted within the clan, and the care given them allowed the prolonged survival of such individuals. These early cases of "social security" go back to the origins of man, some

600,000 years ago, and are attested at least until the Neolithic, in France at least. Cases of care of individuals by the group have been found outside Europe too. For example, a *Homo erectus* skeleton was found on the island of Java, Indonesia, with a completely healed femur. This individual survived the injury thanks to the solidarity of his kin.

At that time, life was rare and precious. Survival of the group relied in part on the mutual support of the weakest—a concept largely forgotten in our so-called "modern" societies. In prehistoric times, unity was power, and so were numbers.[1]

## Note

1. See P. Charlier, "Existait-il une prise en charge des individus infirmes préhistoriques?," *Medicina nei Secoli*, 18/2, 2006, pp. 399–420.

# A PREHISTORIC AMPUTATION

A Neolithic Amputation from Buthiers-Boulancourt

In 2005, a Neolithic skeleton was discovered in Buthiers-Boulancourt, in Seine-et-Marne, forty-four miles (70 km) southeast of Paris. Around 4900–4700 BC, this region was occupied by communities practicing agriculture and pastoralism; several houses and pottery fragments dating to this period were found in the vicinity, as well as a few graves and a cremation site. All this suggests that the site had been lived in for a long time. The grave excavated in 2005 was a so-called "prestigious" burial, belonging to an important person. Indeed, a magnificent flint tool about eight inches (20 cm) long lay by the side of the skeleton, along with the bones of some animals that had probably been sacrificed and buried with the deceased. Overall, the bones were quite well preserved.

The main interest of this discovery lies in the individual's left arm. The distal part of the left humerus had been amputated, so that this person no longer had an elbow or forearm. Following a micro-radiological study, it was clear that this was neither a congenital malformation, nor a trauma resulting from an accident, nor even a postmortem break. Examination of the skeleton did not reveal any other traumatic injuries. This was clearly an intentional surgical act. The doctor was skilful and the patient robust. The cut is clean, as is the healing, for no trace of infection was found around the amputated bone. No trace, either, was found of any heat treatment, so it seems that the wound was not cauterized. And the patient did not suffer any massive hemorrhagic complications, since he survived. The practitioner who performed this surgery demands our respect when we know the techniques and means available at the time. The only remaining unknown is the reason for this amputation. Notwithstanding detailed analyses, it has been impossible to determine what this patient suffered from before the intervention (a tumor, necrosis, infection or other pathology?).

This discovery proves that 7,000 years ago, our distant ancestors had good medical knowledge (a fact we already knew because of trepanning, for example, which has been practiced since the Neolithic). Apart from the surgical act itself, the practitioner of the time took good care of the wound and ensured its healthy healing. The operation was successful, since the patient survived and was able to regain his place within his community. This amputation is not an isolated case in archaeology: other skeletons showing signs of amputation have been found in Europe, but they date to more recent periods (mainly from Roman times). The Buthiers-Boulancourt skeleton is an exceptional case because it is, to the best of our knowledge, the most ancient case of human amputation known to date.[1]

## Note

1. See C. Buquet-Marion, P. Charlier, A. Samzun, "A Possible Early Neolithic Amputation at Buthiers-Boulancourt (Seine-et-Marne), France," *Antiquity*, 322, 2009, p. 83.

# II

## ANTIQUITY

# THE STORY OF THE MUMMY

The Proto-dynastic Egyptian Mummy of an Infant
with Malaria

This case was offered to us by Raffaella Bianucci, an Italian scientist who was trying to establish the presence of malaria in Proto-dynastic Egypt, in other words on mummies dating back to between 5000 and 3000 BC. The key feature of mummies from this period is that they are mostly natural. The process is caused by the dry environment, which spontaneously desiccates bodies deposited in the sand. Some were well-preserved, others turned to dust when they were discovered or transported away from the burial site. Later mummification practices of the Egyptians would only perfect what nature was already doing quite adequately on its own.

With a team of a dozen French and Italian researchers (including one specialist from the Pasteur Institute in Lille), we sought to determine whether the extremely well-preserved mummy of a child from the collections of the Egyptian Museum in Turin contained the malaria parasite. Samples of six microns were taken from the mummy and exposed to antibodies against the antigens of *plasmodium*, the pathogen of this parasitic disease. And, surprisingly, the antibodies still reacted, several thousand years later. In parallel, the same method was applied on negative specimens, to be quite sure that there were no false readings. Once the antibodies were revealed, quantification was possible. Analysis revealed that this young patient was indeed suffering from malaria, though it was impossible to tell if the disease had caused the death of the child.

The importance of this experimental research is to have established scientifically the presence of malaria in that region, at that time. We certainly suspected its existence, but the scientific community had no tangible evidence. The most "recent" evidence, in an identical chrono-cultural context, dated to the Old/Middle Kingdom, in other words between 1,000 and 1,500 years later.

From the technological point of view, this research was interesting because it allowed us to work on particularly ancient and deteriorated human remains, and to improve our knowledge of this disease. It would, in the future, be interesting to sequence our patient's *plasmodium* to find out whether the genetic heritage of this infectious agent has changed since that time. Were the clinical symptoms of malaria in those distant times perhaps also different from those of today's disease?[1]

### Note

1. See R. Bianucci, G. Mattutino, R. Lallo, P. Charlier, H. Jouin-Spriet, A. Peluso, T. Higham, C. Torre, E. Rabino Massa, "Immunological Evidence of *Plasmodium Falciparum* Infection in an Egyptian Child Mummy from the Early Dynastic Period," *Journal of Archaeological Science*, 35, 2008, pp. 1880–1885.

# 4

## RETURN OF THE MUMMY

### Tutankhamun's Fetuses

In an article in the *American Journal of Roentgenology*, Zahi Hawass, the then-Egyptian Minister of Antiquities, and several osteoarchaeologists published their radiographic study of the fetuses of Tutankhamun. They are two stillborn infants from the union of Tutankhamun and his wife Ankhesenamun, who had been embalmed and placed in their father's tomb when he died.

According to Zahi Hawass and his team, the radiography showed two deformed fetuses. One suffered from Sprengel deformity, with anomalies at the shoulder and on the spinal column. For the other, the article said that it was simply extremely premature. According to the authors, the infants were twins who died at the same time.

We took another look at the study of these radiographs—without having examined the bodies themselves, but with a forensic eye. Divergent opinions quickly emerged regarding their study. Firstly, the two infants did not have the same genetic heritage. It was 99.7 percent identical, but not 100 percent, as should have been the case. Therefore they were not real twins, but at best false twins, or simply brother and sister who followed each other in time. Unfortunately, nothing prevents a woman from miscarrying repeatedly.

Secondly, by studying the radiographs, another hypothesis seemed tenable. It was possible that one of the children was not deformed, but had died *in utero*, and was expelled later. The fetus would then have turned into a "macerated fetus"; that is to say that it would have started to decompose in its mother's belly. The anomalies visible were probably linked to the deterioration of the body which, deprived of tone, would have become desiccated and deformed.

This forensic review of the fetuses of Tutankhamun shows that it is difficult to diagnose deformities on such young bodies, which may have deteriorated subsequently through embalming.[1]

### Note

1. See P. Charlier, S. Khung-Savatovsky, I. Huynh-Charlier, "Forensic and Pathology Remarks Concerning the Mummified Fetuses of King Tutankhamun," *American Journal of Roentgenology*, 198/6, 2012, pp. 629 ff.

# 5

## ET IN ARGOLIDE EGO

Earthquake Victims in Midea, Greece,
in the 10th Century BC

Is it possible to distinguish between a broken bone (fracture) at the moment of death, as a result of an earthquake, tremor, or violent burial, and ancient bones broken during the course of their long existence underground?

All that was needed were some suitable skeletons. After appealing to the directors of the archaeological institutes in Greece and Italy, Mr. Paul Åström, the former director of the Swedish Institute at Athens, in Greece, and Ms. Ann-Lise Schällin, the director at the time, found the ideal sample: in their collections they had skeletons from Midea, in Argos, and offered me the chance to study them. In the stores of the Museum of Nafplion (an ancient Ottoman building on the main square), I examined two skeletons. The first was that of a baby (less than one year old) whose particularly fragile bones were intact. This immature individual had been found in the ruins of a Mycenaean house that fell down around 1700 BC. If this baby had died due to the collapse of the house, it would have presented serious traumatic injuries. Thus, the archaeological data and the absence of any fractures together indicated that this infant had been buried in the destroyed layer of the building, but the cause of death remains unknown.

At the time of the excavation, the Swedes had found the body of another individual nearby: a hunched-up adult in the collapsed layer of the same house. Unlike the infant, he greatly resembled the victim of an earthquake. Indeed, the study of this skeleton revealed quite specific traumatic injuries that can be seen in contemporary forensic cases, such as the earthquakes in Algeria, Japan, and Afghanistan. When a ceiling caves in, for example, we know that particular parts of the body are most often affected. When a building collapses, people tend to hunch over instinctively, put themselves in a fetal position, or squat down to protect themselves. At the moment of being crushed, these positions lead to the dislocation of the spine, either at the junction between the lumbar vertebrae and the sacrum, or at the junction between the thoracic and lumbar vertebrae. The same goes for fractures of the petrous temporal bone, at the base of the cranium (this is a dense bone that does not normally fracture when a body is buried for a long time). Another fracture that is typical of being crushed occurs on the body of the scapula (shoulder bone), just under the glenoid cavity—in other words, the part that articulates with the head of the humerus (upper arm bone).

All these classic clinical cases in contemporary medical and surgical publications are the result of earthquakes and other catastrophes, and accidents involving crushing. Similar injuries were found on the second skeleton, and so the fractures must have been due to the violent burial of the person in catastrophic circumstances, and not as a result of a prolonged period underground. This kind of archaeological experimentation allows us to extrapolate from contemporary skeletons recovered during forensic investigations and to identify similar diagnostic criteria in ancient skeletal remains.[1]

## Note

1. See P. Charlier, O. Ferrant, I. Huynh-Charlier, A. I. Sundström, A. L. Schällin, M. Durigon, G. Lorin de La Grandmaison, "Diagnostic différentiel de fractures osseuses d'écrasement/enfouissement *peri-mortem* et de fragilisation osseuse *post mortem*: comparaison de données ostéo-archéologiques et anthropologiques médico-légales," *Journal de médecine légale droit médical*, 51/6, 2008, pp. 301–320.

# 6

## URBI ET ORBI

A Case of Down Syndrome in the Rome of Romulus
and Remus (9th–6th centuries BC)

During archaeological excavations in Rome in the early 20th century, the skeleton of a child was found. Nothing unusual so far, except that the skeleton was discovered on the site of the Roman forum, right in the center of the town, in the foundations of the statue of the Emperor Domitian, who ruled in the 1st century AD. This detail would give the skeleton its name (*Equus domitiani II*); today, it is kept in the stores of the town's archaeological department.

Since its discovery, this skeleton had never been examined, even though its cranium, which was at the very least "strange," greatly intrigued the conservators. . . . We examined this skeleton of a young girl aged between nine and fourteen, and noted that there was a disparity between her dental age (age estimated on tooth eruption), her age by stature (the height of an individual), and the age of the bone (age estimated on the disappearance of growth cartilage). Not only was the face unusual, but the rest of the skeleton presented anomalies: one metacarpal shorter than the others, supernumerary ribs (more than the normal twelve on each side of the thorax), additional sutures on the cranium, and an abnormal pelvis.

This set of anomalies meant that we could diagnose Down syndrome unambiguously. But the terrible thing was that this child had been killed with an axe blow on the head (right parietal bone). One speaks of "trauma on fresh bone" when the skin, blood, and collagen were still present at the moment of death (in other words the fracture on the cranium is not due to the wear and tear of time, or to archaeological excavations). The question was to understand whether this child had been sacrificed ritually, because she carried the "evil eye," or in order to remove an "unnecessary mouth" in this chrono-cultural context.

Even though we cannot provide a definitive answer, this young girl was probably sacrificed to a divinity (the ritual context of the location seems to have been confirmed by recent excavations). When the body was interred, between the 9th and 6th centuries BC and therefore well before the construction of the Forum and the existence of Imperial Rome, this location was outside the town and was used only for religious rituals. At that time, Rome was only a village on a hillside, and sacrifices were made at the bottom of the hill, in the marshes that surrounded the town. After the sacrifices, the bodies were either buried immediately, or thrown into the nearby marshes. By an accident of history, with the growth and remodeling of Rome over the centuries, the marshes were dried out, and the body of the young girl happened to be buried several feet under the statue of Domitian on his horse, right in the center of the town that dominated the antique world.

Other, slightly later, skeletons have been exhumed a few feet away from there at the foot of the Carcer Tullianum, the Mamertine prison in which such people as Jugurtha, Catilina, Vercingetorix, and, closer to our time, Saint Paul were incarcerated. Among these skeletons, a male individual was found with this hands tied behind his back; he too had probably been sacrificed or executed.[1]

## Note

1. See P. Charlier, "Ce que la paléopathologie révèle du statut des sujets malformés dans l'Antiquité gréco-romaine," *La Revue du praticien*, 54/8, 2004, pp. 921–925.

# 7

# BOULEVARD OF BONES

The Etruscan-Celtic Necropolises of Monte Bibele
and Monterenzio Vecchia (3rd Century BC)

Monte Bibele and Monterenzio Vecchia, close to Bologna, Italy, are two necropolises spanning the 4th to 2nd centuries BC. The interest here lay in making a complete study of each and then comparing them. But Monte Bibele had already been well-studied, and of the 300 graves on the site, the latest archeological excavation seasons had found only one unexplored burial. Monterenzio Vecchia is a smaller site, but much richer archaeologically, with around forty graves. Due to my research requirements, I was able to participate in all the excavation seasons as well as study the skeletons *in situ*. This was real field osteoarchaeology, which meant that skeletal anomalies could be diagnosed as soon as the bones were exposed.

Comparison of these two partially contemporary burial sites provided the possibility of reconstructing the daily life of the inhabitants. The populations found in both necropolises were Boii, an Etrusco-Celtic ethnic group, which was often at war with the Latins in Rome.[1]

The various social classes of Boïens were present at both sites. Skeletons from the lower classes were distinguished from those of the aristocracy by the presence of different illnesses. Notably, those from the aristocracy had more caries, linked to the consumption of fast sugars (honey), and various fractures or wounds from cutting weapons, such as swords, that bear witness to the participation of certain individuals in bellicose activities.

Thanks to this necropolis, a new anthropological phenomenon has been described—"solidified putrefaction fluid," which presents in the form of a reddish deposit on the inside of the cranial cavity. It is what remains of a completely decomposed, skeletonized body. This fluid collects in low areas, mainly the bottom of the cranial cavity, which acts almost like a cup. Sometimes it also accumulates on the surface of bones, particularly the pelvis and long bones, the extended shape of which allows the fluid to be preserved and become calcified over time. It can then be studied under the microscope. Putrefaction fluid is extremely viscous and often adheres to the surface of bones, though it can also be found in the bottom of the grave, on the sides of the sarcophagus or coffin.

This fluid was found on many of the crania from Monte Bibele and Monterenzio Vecchia. Examination under a microscope revealed some cellular elements and remains of cloth, for, as a body decomposes, the clothes of the deceased also decompose, along with any accompanying funerary offerings of perishable materials. Red blood cells can also be found (sometimes with parasites—malaria, for example), and fragments of hair, which allow the hair color of the subject under study to be determined. With the microscopic analysis of this fluid, a skeleton can provide researchers with considerable information. Additional analysis allows large sections of the deceased's life to be reconstructed.

Archaeologists knew about this type of reddish liquid on bones, but, as it was considered to be dirt, it was cleaned away, thereby destroying precious information. Following the description of "solidified putrefaction fluid" in the early 2000s, its usefulness was quickly recognized by forensic experts. Henceforth, microscopic studies of this "fluid" have of course been carried out in archaeology, as well as in forensic anthropology, where it has become part of standard procedure. Without knowing it, the dead of Monte Bibele and Monterenzio Vecchia are helping to resolve criminal enquiries of our times.[2]

## Notes

1. This is known principally from Titus Livius (Livy) (39.2), who tells of conflicts between the Latins and Boii during the construction of the Via Flaminia minor, which ran from Bologna to Arezzo and passed across the territories of the Boii, close to Monte Bibele and Monterenzio Vecchia. In the Monterenzio museum there is a Boïen cranium that is cut in two lengthwise by a sword, probably Roman, with a very clean section which, presumably, must have led to immediate death.

2. See P. Charlier, P. Georges, F. Bouchet, I. Huynh-Charlier, R. Carlier, V. Mazel, P. Richardin, L. Brun, J. Blondiaux, G. Lorin de la Grandmaison, "The Microscopic (Optical and SEM) Examination of Putrefaction Fluid Deposits (PFD). Potential Interest in Forensic Anthropology," *Virchows Archiv*, 453/4, 2008, pp. 377–386. See also P. Charlier, *Ostéo-archéologie de deux nécropoles étrusco-celtiques: Monte Bibele et Monterenzio Vecchia (Bologne, Italie). Reconstitution d'une pathocénose à l'échelle de la vallée de l'Idice*, PhD thesis from the École pratique des hautes études, IV$^e$ section, Sciences historiques et philologiques, Paris, 2005.

# 8

# OTHER PEOPLE'S TASTE

Representing Deformity in Antiquity

Between the 3rd and 1st centuries BC, in Hellenistic times, in the town of Smyrna (today's Izmir, in Turkey), there was a tradition of making terra-cotta representations of "comic faces." These terra-cottas, measuring around two inches (5 cm), sometimes known as "grotesques," are not well known. Where they intended for some sort of entertainment? Did they represent theatrical actors? Or did they show types of patients or diseases for use in the school of medicine in Smyrna, which was fairly important in antiquity? We do not know. The interested reader can see some in Paris, in the Louvre Museum, in Brussels at the Cinquatenaire Museum, as well as in the Metropolitan Museum in New York, for example.

One day, a new case was presented to me, representing an individual with facial paralysis. Unlike the statuettes from the same period, the face is clearly asymmetrical. Detailed inspection showed that it was evidently not a mistake made by the craftsman; the anatomical accuracy and the careful execution are quite remarkable: the face was indeed represented as it really was, the craftsman seems to have worked with a living model. The statuette deliberately reproduces the asymmetry of the neck and face. Another statuette, also from Smyrna, represents a Down syndrome child, with all the features of the syndrome appearing in fine detail. Accordingly, the question arises of why an artist took the time to represent two cases of "deformation" or "malformation" of the face. In order to understand the reasons better, one has to look at how deformation and malformation were seen in antiquity.

During archaic, classical Greek antiquity, as well as in Rome during the Republic, the malformed or deformed were traditionally eliminated. They represented the "evil eye" because they were an aberration of nature, because they were a negative message sent by the gods. A change occurred during the Hellenistic period in Greece and the Imperial period in Rome. Both anatomical knowledge and medicine were progressing. Previously, a child born with six toes had been considered deformed. Now, it could be operated on, and the deformity, in any case benign, disappeared. Mentalities had changed, "monsters"—as they were though of at the time—were no longer systematically eliminated.

In imperial Roman times, the "monster" in fact became a source of prestige and entertainment. In this new chrono-cultural context, to own a monster was to own a curiosity of nature, therefore a precious possession. In Rome, there were actual "monster markets" where, for a small fortune, one could buy malformed individuals. When the rapid transit railway line was being built between Rome and Naples, a necropolis was found, near the Via Lucrezia Romana, with more than a hundred Roman slaves probably belonging to a nearby Roman villa. Its owner must have been rich and powerful, for in this cemetery several malformed individuals were found. It is not impossible that they were "breeding" monsters in this villa, through hybridization or by selection.

These human "monsters" served the same purpose as works of art do today. In the Roman Empire, a powerful man receiving his guests for a banquet would show his "monsters," as in the 18th century a parvenu liked to exhibit a Fragonard. If the "monsters" were alive, they danced (the infamous "dance of the monsters"), participated in the banquet, entertained the guests and so on. If they were dead, their remains were exhibited for all to see, preserved in honey, or as mounted skeletons. And the rarer the "monster," the greater the prestige of the owner. To maintain the "herd" of the master, there was no hesitation in coupling the "monsters" with each other in order to obtain new ones, even to amputate or cripple those judged not to be deformed enough!

It was also during this period that deformed people entered into anatomical collections, as well as into "cabinets of curiosities." Their bodies and skeletons were beginning to be collected for study and also to show them to enthusiasts. Pliny the Elder, in volume VII of his *Natural History*, tells us of these cabinets of curiosities, in which such "monsters" are displayed: "In the reign of Augustus, there were two persons, Posio and Secundilla by name, who were half a foot taller than him [the nine-foot nine-inch tall Gabbarus]; their bodies have been preserved as objects of curiosity in the museum of the Sallustian family [ . . . ]. We learn from Varro that Manius Maximus and M. Tullius, members of our equestrian order, were only two cubits in height; and I have myself seen them, preserved in their coffins."[1] Again in his *Natural History*, Pliny the Elder mentions the particular care taken of some of them: "It was thought proper in Egypt to rear a human monster, that had two additional eyes in the back part of the head; it could not see with them, however."[2] The question of the "monsters" nagged at Christian thinkers. Thus, Saint Augustine asked himself: When twins are born with joined bodies—in other words, a body with two heads—should one baptize one or two souls?

If the rich could afford to have skeletons of "monsters" to entertain themselves and to show to their illustrious guests, it was not the case for more modest people, who fell back on reproductions in terra-cotta. These statues were not artworks based on imagination but on representations of reality. Of course, the sculptor sometimes exaggerated: some anatomical elements were represented abnormally, but modern medical knowledge allows us to separate anatomical veracity from artistic exaggeration. Nevertheless, some representations from that time were genuine medical cases, and not "monstrosities" at all. Thus, among these "grotesques," one statuette might represent a case of tetanus, another a case of rickets, and so on.

These objects also raise questions about artistic perception. When one looks at an artwork that might appear strange to us, it is not necessarily representing a disease. It is important to make an accurate diagnosis before creating risky hypotheses. From antiquity we have numerous texts evoking medical cases, corroborated or not by artifacts made by craftsmen. Yet deformities shown on such artifacts might be due to the clumsiness of the artist, or there could equally have been an attempt at imagination, or even perhaps a particular message by the sculptor. In the past, faulty diagnoses have been made by overzealous archaeologists and doctors who saw diseases everywhere. Comparison with some present-day cases (Orthodox ex-votos in Greece, and Catholic ones in southern Italy, for example) allows us to reassess some diagnoses. Let us cite a few examples. During Roman, Gallo-Roman, Greek, and Etruscan antiquity, sick people who went to therapeutic sanctuaries left either texts to give thanks for being healed, or ex-votos. Many examples are found representing breasts, hands, phalluses, eyes, ears, etc. The act of depositing an ex-voto in the form of an ear does not necessarily mean that one was cured of deafness—it could equally be an invocation to the divinity to *hear* the prayer; an ex-voto in the form of an eye could be to ask it to *cast its gaze* on the patient; a foot signifies that one has made the effort to *walk* all the way to the sanctuary; to offer a phallus signifies that one wishes for a child, not necessarily that one wishes to be cured of an STD. . . . Still in this domain, what can one say about an ancient ex-voto representing a breast with its end crushed? Contrary to what one might have thought, it is not necessarily a representation of breast cancer, but could be a "misfired piece," a "defective" ex-voto, as we would say today, that, instead of being thrown away, was sold cheaply to someone who could not afford to buy a good-quality one. Nearer to us, some ex-votos have been found at the headwaters of the Seine. They were made of wood and the artist had to deal with the demands of the materials. Some ex-votos were twisted, and it was thought for a long time that they were representations of rickets, which is in all likelihood incorrect: the artist simply carved an ex-voto in a thin, twisted branch. When, at the beginning of the 20th century, pilgrims coming to Lourdes bought souvenirs, often made by local artisans, some occasionally showed a slight imperfection (a squint, asymmetry, etc.). This does not mean that the Virgin Mary was cross-eyed. In other words, one must not see diseases everywhere.

Another interesting case is that of the representation of phimosis. When looking at Antique statues, most men are not circumcised: only slaves and some strangers were. If one examines these Antique Greek and Roman statues carefully, one sees that the foreskin is tight across the glans penis. For a long time it was thought that this was a representation of phimosis and numerous articles were published about this in the past. But this is not the representation of a disease, it is simply an artistic code. If all Greek and Roman youths had been afflicted with phimosis, classical civilizations would have disappeared in one generation! In classical Antique statuary, the representation of the face did not always allow the origin of the model to be determined. The origin of the individual could be transferred to the genitals. With this pseudo-phimosis, and the absence of circumcision, the artist specified the Greek or Roman origin of the subject of the sculpture.

These representations of "deformity" help us to understand better the period in which they were made. They are also of great scientific interest. Regarding the statuette with the asymmetrical face, it is clearly a case of facial paralysis. However, such paralysis is muscular and temporary, and completely invisible on a skeleton. For facial paralysis to be detectable on the bones, it has to be chronic, with an asymmetry between the left and right parts of the cranium. Such a case was found in the necropolis of the Via Lucrezia Romana mentioned above. The chronic cranial asymmetry was confirmed by a significant tartar deposit (almost three-quarters of an inch [2 cm] thick!) on only one side of the jaw. Facial paralysis is often accompanied by more abundant secretion of saliva, and sometimes by paralysis of the tongue.

Sometimes a sculpture or an ancient text allows a fairly accurate diagnosis to be made of something that would be completely invisible on a skeleton, and thereby helps to complete the global tableau of the state of health of past populations.[3]

## Notes

1. Pliny the Elder, *The Natural History*, 7, 16, translated from the Latin by John Bostock, http://www.perseus.tufts.edu/hopper/text?doc=Perseus%3Atext%3A 1999.02.0137%3Abook%3D7%3Achapter%3D16.

2. Ibid., 11, 113, p. 579.

3. See P. Charlier, "Un nouveau cas de paralysie faciale sur une terre-cuite smyrniote hellénistique. Icono-diagnostic et paléopathologie des paralysies facials," *Histoire des sciences médicales*, 46/1, 2007, pp. 49–60 and *ibid., Les Monstres humains dans l'Antiquité. Analyse paléopathologique*, Paris, Fayard, 2008.

# 9

## THE FIRE OF GOD

Greek Cremations in Romania (3rd Century BC)

Thanks to an old friend, Alexandre Baralis, I was able to work on Greek cremations from the archaeological site of Orgame (Argamum), on the shores of the Black Sea in Romania. On a promontory overlooking the delta of the Danube was one of the most remote Greek colonies on the Black Sea. The surrounding wetlands produce a surreal landscape, and vertical cliffs plunge into the intense blue Danube flowing below. Far away, on the opposite bank, the hills of Ukraine can be discerned. . . . The nearest town to the archaeological site is Jurilovca, six miles (10 km) away, and at the time, the only accommodation available to the archaeologists was with a Lippovan Russian community.

Orgame was founded on the majestic rocky cliff top. An important and prosperous town, it traded all around the Black Sea, but mostly with the Crimea. They had wheat and Baltic amber, which was traded down the Danube. One can still see the town's ruined monumental gates, Greek, Roman and Byzantine houses, as well as an early Christian basilica that bears witness to the fact that the town was occupied until the 9th century AD, after which the inhabitants abandoned it. There were probably multiple causes for this abandonment, such as the harbor silting up, depletion of the trade route, barbarian raids, and so on.

But let us return to the Greek period. On the outskirts of the town was the "camp of the dead," currently being excavated by Vasilica Lungu. In the center is a majestic tumulus several dozen yards wide, the *Heroon*—the hero's tomb—in other words the grave of the first person who came from Greece in the 8th century BC to establish himself here and who was honored with a monumental tomb. Having become the mythical founder of the town, all its inhabitants then wanted to be buried as close to him as possible.

This Greek colony also had a *necromanteion*, situated outside the town. Such sanctuaries served to ask questions of the dead and to speak to the deceased of one's family. The layout of a *necromanteion* is a small labyrinth leading one along a symbolic passage ending in a well, at the bottom of which is a vaulted chamber. Here, with the help of abundant smoke, one enters into contact with the dead. At the end of this journey, after a purification ritual, one would return to the town. The fact that Orgame had a *necromanteion* indicates that mystery cults were being practiced there in antiquity, even though it is cruder than those found in mainland Greece, such as at Mantinea. Interestingly, both these *necromanteion* are in similar locations on rocky promontories, far from the town and its houses, and close to swamps.

Laetitia Laquay and I wanted to understand the cremation ritual of those Greek colonists from the 7th to 5th centuries BC. We quickly realized that the cremation ritual was of the Homeric type—in other words, the 8th-century founder of the town had been honored by a funeral inspired by the cremations of heroes in the *Iliad*.[1] And so, by analogy, down the centuries, all the inhabitants practiced the same ritual and had themselves incinerated, then buried around the main tumulus, thus attracting honor to themselves by proximity. However, this type of cremation is typically Greek. The Greek colonists, even on the Black Sea borders, never practiced local rituals nor integrated local funeral practices. When they established themselves on the shores of the Danube, they also brought their funerary traditions, and never changed them. The hero's tumulus contained offerings of large animals and ritually broken amphorae arranged in circles around him. The bone fragments found in the graves around the central tumulus are too fragmented to be able to distinguish between Greek bones and those of the local Hellenized population. The only certainty is the homogeneity of the rites, down the centuries, in honor of the founding hero.[2]

## Notes

1. See Chapter 10, below.
2. See L. Laquay, D. Favier, G. F. Jeannel, M. Patou-Mathis, J. Poupon, S. Thiébault, A. Baralis, V. Lungu, P. Charlier, "Étude archéo-anthropologique des crémations de l'Hérôon d'Orgamé (Roumanie, troisième quart du VIIe siècle avant notre ère)," in P. Charlier, D. Gourevitch (eds), *Quatrième Colloque international de pathographie (Saint-Jean-de-Côle, 2011)*, Paris, De Boccard, 2013, pp. 61–67.

# 10

# A HERO OF OUR TIME

## A Greek Cremation in the Louvre Museum

In the Louvre Museum there are some very interesting bronze statues that are worth a visit, particularly for anyone interested in Greek funerary rites. This venerable institution preserves innumerable funerary vases of multiple forms. For example, the Department of Greek, Etruscan, and Roman Antiquities displays a hydria that—as its name suggests—was used to hold water, and that had been "recycled" into a funerary urn in which there are still a few fragments of bone. Under the aegis of Sophie Deschamps, conservator in that department, I became interested in another very interesting piece containing some human remains.

The vase presents in the shape of a bronze cooking pot, twelve inches (31 cm) in diameter by almost eight inches (20 cm) high.[1] It had been found during excavations near Athens in the 19th century, in a small semicircular cavity cut into stone, covered by a small tumulus. Soon after, it was acquired by the Louvre Museum. Its main interest lies in the inscription: "The Athenians give prizes to those who have fallen in war." Therefore, the pot contained the remains of a soldier who died during a battle against the Persians, in the 5th century BC. Perhaps he had been at the battle of Marathon, or of Salamis, or Plataea. . . . At his death, the body was first incinerated, then the ashes were placed in this vessel (known as a *lebes*) and finally buried. Almost two kilograms of human remains were found in this vessel, consisting of teeth, pieces of phalanges, pelvic bones, vertebrae, long bones, and numerous unidentified fragments.

The study of the remains from the pot showed that they belonged to a single young adult. In the fire, the fusion between metal and the fat of the individual formed a precipitate, the analysis of which showed that when the soldier was cremated his body had been accompanied by iron and copper from his weapons and other precious objects (e.g. fibulae, rings). No animal bones were found, but wood—olive wood, to be more precise—was also identified. This would either have been wood from the funeral pyre, or from a wooden object placed with the remains of the deceased.

The cremation ritual of our individual is in every detail like that of Patrocles or Hector, as described by Homer in the *Iliad*:

> Those who were about the dead heaped up wood and built a pyre a hundred feet this way and that; then they laid the dead all sorrowfully upon the top of it. They flayed and dressed many fat sheep and oxen before the pyre, and Achilles took fat from all of them and wrapped the body therein from head to foot, heaping the flayed carcases all round it. Against the bier he leaned two-handled jars of honey and unguents; four proud horses did he then cast upon the pyre, groaning the while he did so. The dead hero had had house-dogs; two of them did Achilles slay and threw upon the pyre; he also put twelve brave sons of noble Trojans to the sword and laid them with the rest, for he was full of bitterness and fury. Then he committed all to the resistless and devouring might of the fire . . . [The next day the Greeks collected the remains of the hero]. First they poured red wine upon the thick layer of ashes and quenched the fire. With many tears they singled out the whitened bones of their loved comrade and laid them within a golden urn in two layers of fat: they then covered the urn with a linen cloth and took it inside the tent. They marked off the circle where the barrow should be, made a foundation for it about the pyre, and forthwith heaped up the earth. When they had thus raised a mound they went away.[2]

This ritual, appropriate for the heroes of Greek antiquity, was already ancient in the 5th century BC, if one considers that the *Iliad* dates to the 8th century BC. The point of this type of funerary practice was to make a hero of the deceased by giving him a ceremony akin to that of mythological heroes. It was not a ritual offered to a simple "soldier," who generally had to be satisfied with a grave or a collective pyre. Our individual must have enjoyed a certain rank in the military hierarchy, and had sufficient financial means to buy the bronze cooking pot at the very least. Taken together, the scientific and literary information allows us to learn much about the individual under examination, despite his very fragmented remains.

Such Homeric rituals would continue until the Roman era, when military men, aristocrats, and wealthy educated figures would choose this type of funeral to integrate themselves, *post mortem*, with the heroes of the *Iliad*, they who never die. . . . [3]

## Notes

1. BR 2590 in the museum inventory. On permanent display in the salle des Bronzes.

2. Homer, *Iliad*, vol. IV, XXIII—160/250, translated from the Greek by Samuel Butler, *The Iliad of Homer, Rendered into English Prose* (1898). For Hector's funeral, see *ibid.*, XXIV—782/805.

3. See P. Charlier, J. Poupon, M. Goubard, S. Descamps, "'In This Way They Held Funeral for Horse-Taming Hector': a Greek Cremation Reflects Homeric Ritual," in L.A. Schepartz, S.C. Fox, C. Bourbou (eds), *New Directions in the Skeletal Biology of Greece*, Athens, American School of Classical Studies at Athens, 2009, pp. 49–56.

# 11

# DRUNKEN OFFENSE

A Case of Alcoholism in Antiquity

This scene happens in the archaeological museum of Rethymnon in Crete. I was patiently waiting to be given access to a skeleton from the site of Eleftherna in order to study it, when, walking through the deserted halls, I came to a halt in front of an ancient stele bearing an incomplete inscription. So far, this was hardly unexpected in such a place, except that the text on this stone, dating to the 6th century BC, was devoted to problems linked with drunkenness in public places. This fairly short edict forbade the consumption of alcohol in certain parts of the town and described the signs of drunkenness very succinctly. Here was an illuminating case of daily life in ancient Greece, all the more so since it is currently virtually impossible to detect a state of alcoholism on a skeleton. . . .

Clarisse Prêtre, a philologist friend, made as faithful a translation as possible of this inscription. The idea was to find out to which sanctuary it belonged, as well as why it was necessary to stamp out drunkenness. We also investigated whether other sources described this kind of behavior. Several texts from the Greco-Roman period indeed state that one was not allowed to be drunk on public roads. Drunkenness was authorized only at particular times, notably among the young, during initiation ceremonies or "rites of passage." At Delphi, for example, it was forbidden to bring alcohol into certain parts of the sanctuary.

A total of three texts, covering three centuries of history, deal with drunkenness on public roads. Admittedly, this is not much, and a comparison through time seems risky. Nevertheless, it demonstrates the recurrence of the problem, and that it was, already, condemned by a segment of society. Numerous classical authors wrote "hygienist" texts warning against the dangers of wine and its consequences: dizziness and so on. Others advised its consumption for its therapeutic virtues. . . . *In vino veritas?*[1]

## Note

1. See P. Charlier, C. Prêtre, "Alcoholism in Antiquity: from Repression to Therapy," in H. Perdicoyianni-Paléologou (ed.), *The Concept of Madness from Homer to Byzantium: History and Aspects*, Amsterdam, Supplementi di Lexis, Adolf Hakkert, 2016, pp. 33 ff.

# 12

## ANCIENT MIRACLES

Accounts of Divine Cures in Greco-Roman Antiquity

Still with the philologist Clarisse Prêtre, we were able to work on accounts of miraculous cures in Greco-Roman antiquity. To heal themselves, some sick people preferred to rely on the gods, such as Asclepius, Theos Hypsistos, Poseidon, Apollo, etc., rather than on doctors of the Hippocratic tradition. In such cases, patients went to a therapeutic sanctuary where they followed a process that today would be considered a ritual cure. By staying in the sanctuary, patients submitted themselves to a specific diet and conditions of hygiene, sacrificed an animal to the god in question and spent the nights in the *abaton* (a sort of large covered gallery in which the beds were side by side) or in a *tholos* (a circular building in which snakes could wander). There, while asleep, the patient was visited by the divinity and had dreams that were meant to help in healing. On awaking, with the help of the priests, the divine words were interpreted, and a therapeutic process was devised.

As soon as the patient was better, he or she might have a stele sculpted to tell the story. Depending on patients' means, the stele could be large or small, and the inscription more or less detailed. These *iamata*, as they are known, were placed in the sanctuary, and acted as publicity by showing the quality of the care offered. These stelae are particularly interesting because they sometimes constitute proper "medical dossiers," allowing a retrospective diagnosis to be suggested, as well as a better understanding of the medicine of the time. Such *iamata* have been found in Epidaurus in Greece and in many other Greek and Roman sanctuaries. For our work, we chose around fifty texts and analyzed some of the cures from a medical standpoint to see whether the treatment used was effective (founded on relative medical empiricism) or was based on a miracle, or exaggeration. Here we present three of the most representative and instructive cases.

The first is that of Kleo, in the 4th century BC. The stele comes from Epidaurus:

> She had already been pregnant for five years when she came as a suppliant to the god and went to sleep in the innermost sanctuary. As soon as she came out of it and was outside the sanctuary, she gave birth to a boy, who as soon as he was born washed himself from the fountain and walked about with his mother. After being granted this favor she wrote the following inscription on her dedication: "It is not the size of the tablet that deserves admiration, but the divinity, as Kleo was pregnant with child in her womb for five years, until she went to sleep and the divinity restored her to health."[1]

From a medical viewpoint, this story seems fictional and irrational. Such a long human pregnancy does not exist, and no child just come from his mother's belly can perform such feats. . . . Several hypotheses are possible. Perhaps it was an abdominal mass, or an ovarian tumor, which can grow to be several inches and can resemble a pregnancy. There are also pregnancies that, ending abruptly, can be followed by the mummification or even the gradual calcification of the fetus if it has not been expelled (lithopedion), though that does not seem to be the case here.

Another interesting case is that of a voiceless child, still in the 4th century BC in Epidaurus:

> This one came to the sanctuary because of his voice. Having completed the preliminary sacrifices and done what was required, the young man carrying the sacred fire for the god then demanded, looking toward

the father of the child, the promise, if the reason for his coming was acquitted, to make a sacrifice as a payment for his cure within the year. The child suddenly said "I promise." His father, very surprised, asked him to repeat it and he repeated it. Thereafter, he recovered his health.

For this young man, we are probably dealing with the power of suggestion. The stele presents the patient as having "no voice," but without any further detail. The lack of speech could have two causes: a lesion on the vocal chords, or a neurological accident. This young man was probably mute—in other words, he could speak, but, for neurological reasons, he did not do so. The rites of the sanctuary, the emotional control of the voice, and the suggestion of the priests could have played a role in his cure. Unless it was a glottic edema of the vocal chords caused by an infection, or cold, or trauma (overuse of the voice), which was resorbed naturally at the moment when the patient found himself in the sanctuary. Either hypothesis is plausible.

Another case from the same period and location as the previous ones is that of a man cured by a serpent:

He had a toe in bad condition because of an ugly swelling. That day, he had been carried by the servants and he stayed seated on a chair. When he fell asleep, a serpent came out of the *abaton* and healed his foot with its tongue, after which it returned to the *abaton*. He awoke in good health and recounted that in his vision, he thought that a handsome young man had poured a remedy on his toe.

The snake is a symbolic animal very much present in ancient medicine (the caduceus). In antiquity, the therapeutic possibilities afforded by the secretions of some animals were already known. To cure certain skin diseases, dog saliva might be used (a saliva which, as we know today, contains far more leucocytes than human saliva). Serpent saliva was assumed to have active substances, particularly for the skin. It is not impossible, although for this patient, some unguents must have been applied.

*Abatons* referred to the divine, but the use of potions was also practiced, as a stele from Lebena relates, which dates to between the 2nd and 1st centuries BC:

Since I had been coughing non-stop for two years, so much so that I was coughing up bloody and putrid tissue all day long, the god undertook to cure me. He made me eat some rocket, then drink some peppered Italian wine, then starch in hot water, sacred powdered ash in sacred water, an egg with pine resin, and also raw pitch, then iris in honey; then he made me drink quince juice mixed with spurge, eat some apple, then fig with some sacred ash from the altar where sacrifices to the gods are made.

Unfortunately, this stele is incomplete, but it gives an accurate enough idea of the treatment. This patient was given a proper "prescription" and the purge must have been severe. Indeed, rocket has very varied properties (diuretic, aphrodisiac, analgesic); starch also has real therapeutic properties for digestive and intestinal complaints in a broad sense, as well as for head colds; iris mixed with honey acts as a purgative; quinces and apples are known for providing intestinal relief, and when associated with starch make a purgative therapy for the patient realistic. Finally, spurge (euphorbia) is also known for its numerous curative virtues, including as an intestinal purgative that helps evacuations downwards, and spiny spurge with honey can be used for some respiratory illnesses. Figs also have some purgative properties.

Finally, let us cite a case well known in antiquity, that of Hermodikos of Lampascus at Epidaurus in the 4th century BC:

It is as a testimony to your power, Asclepius, that I dedicated this stone that I had lifted, so that the demonstration of your art should be obvious in the eyes of everyone. Indeed, before putting myself in your hands and those of your children, I was stricken by a horrible illness, with a purulent chest and deficient arms. But you, Paean, having persuaded me that this stone could be lifted, you delivered me from the disease.

Lacking more specific indications, we can diagnose a chest infection accompanied by an injury of the brachial plexus with a temporary motor impairment of the upper limbs. But was this compression due to an inflamed edema? To an abscess or a deep hematoma? We do not know; the term "purulent" could be used for all of these clinical situations. Nevertheless, what makes this *iamata* unusual is that it is engraved on the stone that Hermodikos of Lampascus lifted it up after he was cured. It is now in the museum of Epidaurus and weighs a mere 550 pounds(250 kg)!

Reading these *iamata*, it seems that the therapies being practiced in these sanctuaries were based on good medical sense, with particular importance being placed on dietary regimes. The alternating of these treatments with "psychosomatic shocks," rest, and the consumption of a few toxic products could explain cases of real cures. Doctors at the time had academic knowledge (the influence of the environment) but, under the cloak of religion, priests also practiced a form of medicine. Once the patient was cured, when he was about to leave, having had an *iamata* engraved, he had to pay his "honorarium" at the sanctuary (in fact, offerings).

And woe betide anyone who did not comply, like Hermon of Thasos, cured of his total blindness: "Following that, as he did not acquit himself of his medical honorarium, the god made him blind again. So he came back and, after having once more fallen asleep, he regained his health."[2]

## Note

1. Michel Austin, *The Hellenistic World from Alexander to the Roman Conquest: A Selection of Ancient Sources in Translation*, 2nd ed. Cambridge, Cambridge University Press, 2006, p. 269.

2. See C. Prêtre, P. Charlier, *Maladies humaines, thérapies divines. Analyse épigraphique et paléopathologique de textes de guérison grecs*, Lille, Presses universitaires du Septentrion, 2009.

# 13

## DOMAIN OF THE GODS

### Anatomical Ex-votos in Antiquity

In Greco-Roman and even Etruscan antiquity, in order to be cured one had to choose between two main possibilities. One choice was to be examined by a doctor of the Hippocratic school, who made sacrifices to the gods but believed that diseases were linked to the patient's environment and that they could be cured with medicines, regimes, and postures— treatment was sometimes empirical, often experimental, and it is the ancestor of modern medicine. As we have seen above, the patient could also opt for "divine therapy," in other words appeal to the gods of healing. Such a patient would go to therapeutic sanctuaries and ask the divinity or his assistants for a cure. Once in the sanctuary, the patient offered an anatomical ex-voto to the divinity. This ex-voto could come in several forms: a wooden statue, a representation of an organ in terra-cotta, or some perishable material. These ex-votos were offered as much to ask for recovery as to give thanks for being healed.

With my archaeologist and art historian colleagues, I wished to look at these ex-votos with a medical eye to see whether they represented diseased organs with a clearly identifiable pathology, or resulted from the craftsman's lack of skill; being neither a doctor nor an anatomist, he could easily make a mistake. We inventoried numerous ex-votos from French sites, such as those from the museums of Chamalières and Dijon, and from sites in other countries like Musarna (Etruscan ex-votos), Epidaurus (Greece), Rome, etc.

Some of the representations of these ex-votos are very realistic, allowing quite accurate medical diagnoses to be made. For example, a Minoan ex-voto in the archaeological museum of Heraklion represents an edema in a leg, one leg being twice as thick as the other. This illness was represented quite deliberately and could not have been due to the craftsman's carelessness. Another such ex-voto, preserved today in the Louvre Museum, came from Golgoi, an Imperial Roman town on the island of Cyprus; it is in the form of a rebus: one sees a young man with white hair, two eyes next to each other, also painted white, and a left foot with three toes. In fact, this ex-voto represents a polymalformative syndrome (Chediak Higashi syndrome, which combines ectrodactyly—fingers or toes fused together, resembling claws—"silver" hair from a very young age, and albinism of the skin and eyes). This ex-voto was thus made for a patient displaying clinical signs who came to ask the gods to heal him—with little hope of being heard, unfortunately.

Another ex-voto, found in Compiègne in the temple in the forest of Halatte (a large Gallo-Roman therapeutic sanctuary), and today kept in the National Archaeology Museum of Saint-Germain-en-Laye, represents an eye with two pupils. It is a case of a serious malformation, cyclopia. These are generally children who are born with a single eye in the center of their forehead: the two eyes are fused, with two pupils in a single eyeball. This ex-voto is, so far, the only palpable or solid proof of the existence of cyclopia in Greco-Roman antiquity. We know that the disease was present at the time from descriptions, notably by Livy, but no cyclopean skeleton from antiquity has ever been found.

The use of ex-votos was widespread around the whole Mediterranean and in Europe, from the distant past until the dawn of Christianity. Scientific study of these objects allows us to sort between those representing real pathologies and those resulting from the clumsiness of the craftsman, based on scientific criteria. Once sorted, these ex-votos provide information particularly about diseases that leave no trace on the skeleton, such as an inguinal hernia, an exophthalmos (an eye that protrudes excessively from the socket), a tumor, an inflammation, an edema in a limb, and so on. These ex-votos also need to be compared with the ancient texts that have come down to us, some of which describe pathologies. Other than finding a mummy with these sorts of lesions, such ex-votos fill the gap in our understanding of diseases of the soft tissues in past populations, and help to create a better medical record for these ancient periods.[1]

## Note

1. See P. Charlier, "Étude médicale d'ex-voto anatomiques d'Europe occidentale et méditerranéenne," in C. Bobas, C. Evangelidis, T. Milioni, A. Muller (eds), *Croyances populaires. Rites et représentations en Méditerranée Orientale*, Lille, Presses universitaires du Septentrion, 2008, pp. 271–296.

# 14

# MEMORIES FROM THE HOUSE
# OF THE DEAD

The Tortured of Fourni at Delos
(2nd–1st Centuries BC)

As part of some physical anthropology research on violent deaths, I obtained a scholarship to the French School at Athens and went to work on the island of Delos, where, in the 1960s, the French archaeologist Christian Le Roy had made a singular discovery when he exhumed two human skeletons from the cesspit of the house of Fourni. These Delos skeletons would provide a good example, in an archaeological and medical context, of reconstructing how people could be put to death.

Objectively, these two skeletons had no business being there. They were "relegated" to this grave, and throwing the bodies in the latrines meant they were marked by the stamp of infamy—all the more so since the latrines continued to function after their death: the skeletons were deeply covered in excrement. When Christian Le Roy excavated the site, he also found nails in direct contact with the skeletons. In all likelihood, these two adults had been submitted to an *apotympanismos*, in other words a horizontal crucifixion. This was a fairly particular mode of execution, reserved for the lowest social classes, such as slaves, pirates, prostitutes, desecrators of sanctuaries, etc. The process consisted of laying the victim horizontally on a plank and nailing down their wrists and feet. Thus exposed, the victim died slowly of dehydration, sunstroke, respiratory failure, thromboembolic complications (thrombosis linked to immobilization), or even being eaten alive by roaming animals. . . . The two individuals of Delos did not have to wait for death to occur "naturally": one was decapitated and the other received the *coup de grace* with a nail through the femoral artery, leading to a rapid end.

When the skeletons were discovered in the 1960s, the archaeologists were convinced that the victims of this cruel torture were male, and no forensic examination was carried out. Yet, when cleaning some of the bones and examining the pelvic girdles, I was able to discover that they belonged to two women who were less than forty-five years of age when they were put to death. One of the two victims had worn leg irons around the knees for a long time, causing an inflammatory reaction of the bone in contact with them—which suggests that she had been incarcerated for a long time before her execution. The Carbon-14 dating confirmed that this torture occurred between the 2nd and 1st centuries BC.

The most curious thing in this story is that this way of putting people to death was illegal. Indeed, in 426 BC, the city of Athens (Delos was a dependant of Athens) had ordered the "purification" of the island and forbade anyone at all from being buried on the island of Delos. The place was not to be soiled either by blood or death, otherwise disaster would befall the city. All the graves of Delos were emptied, and their contents transferred to the island of Rhenia. From that date onward, no one was allowed to die or to be born on the island of Delos: the dying and women about to give birth were also transferred to Rhenia. If, by misfortune, a corpse landed on the beach, or an inhabitant suffered a heart attack, the body was immediately transferred to a boat, and a purification ceremony was held to efface this contamination. Only a few graves escaped this "purification," notably those on top of which houses had been built, those of hyperborean virgins, semi-goddesses of the cult of Apollo . . . and our two skeletons.

*     *     *

By putting these two women to death on the island of Delos, the inhabitants were breaking the law. The house of Fourni, where this drama unrolled, was situated in the Bay of Fourni, a little apart from the town and port of Delos. According to the bas-reliefs and sculptures found by the archaeologists, the house of Fourni was a building in which "mysteries" occurred, probably the place for meetings of an eastern sect in which the cult of Isis, of Mithra, or of Cybele was practiced. Had our two women defiled the site? But in the case of desecration, they would have been judged by a tribunal of Delos, and their ultimate execution would have been carried out on the island of Rhenia. Who were they? Pirate women? Prostitutes? Witches? Thieves? Most probably, these two women committed an unidentified misdemeanor, and for that, were assassinated outside any legal framework. They were put to death secretly in this house, and the bodies thrown in the cesspit (with the planks) to make them disappear from the world. Why? We do not know. The mystery remains complete . . . and the assassin still runs free.[1]

## Note

1. See P. Charlier, C. Le Roy, C. Keyser, B. Ludes, I. Huynh, "Les suppliciées de Fourni. Étude anthropologique médico-légale de deux squelettes hellénistiques de Délos," *Journal de médecine légale et droit de la santé*, 51/7–8, 2008, pp. 375–385.

# 15

# AN UPSIDE-DOWN BONE . . .

## Pathological Skeletons in Roman
## Romania (1st Century AD)

In the town of Tulcea, Romania, about thirty-one miles (50 km) from Or-game, skeletons from the Roman period are often found when work is carried out on the public highways. Taking advantage of being in the region,[1] I went to the local archaeological museum where there were some recently found skeletons that had not yet been studied in any way, the conservator having no physical anthropologist at his disposal. A male skeleton showed interesting traumatic lesions, notably on the upper limbs, with traces of scarring above the shoulder, and a fractured mandible that had been looked after in a fairly remarkable fashion by a physician. According to the archaeologist, everything points to it being a Roman legionnaire who died in the region.

A second, extremely interesting case, was that of the skeleton of a young woman about twenty-five years old. Examination of the bones showed that her aorta was located on her right side, whereas it is normally found on the left, on the side of the heart. The continual beating of the aorta eventually imprints a mark on the lower thoracic and upper lumbar vertebrae, and slightly flattens the left anterior part of the body of the vertebrae. In some hypertensive patients, these vertebrae can even become concave due to the massive dilation of this large artery.

The pathology of this young woman corresponds to the dextroposition of the aorta, which is a congenital anatomical malformation. Therefore, I endeavored to find out whether this was an isolated lesion or was associated with other anomalies. The study showed that she also had a chronic inflammation of the nasal cavities and the pleura. And finally, the frontal sinuses (in her cranium) were missing. . . . All these clinical indicators suggest Kartagener's syndrome—a congenital defect of the movement of the motile cilia or hairs. These cilia, found on the surface of the respiratory mucous membranes, are indispensable for the movement of mucus. If it stagnates, it provokes chronic infections in the lungs, bronchial tubes, and sinuses. The poor girl must have coughed all the time to clear the mucus obstructing her airways. Patients with Kartagener's syndrome also have atrophied or even absent frontal sinuses, and an inversion of organs (*situs inversus*), the heart and the spleen being on the right side, and the liver on the left side.[2] The last point of interest: the syndrome also causes the subject to be sterile because the vibrating cilia cannot move in the Fallopian tubes of women; the same for the sperm of men.

The lesions on this young woman's bones exactly match this pathology. It is therefore possible to make an accurate diagnosis of the disease, because even though it manifests itself in perishable organs, it also leaves traces on the skeleton. We have published an article that highlights the benefits of a systematic examination for vertebral flattening.[3] Physical anthropologists normally look systematically to see on which side of the lower thoracic and upper lumbar vertebrae this mark is found, thereby showing the placement of the aorta, including on bones that are several million years old. The ancient skeleton of this young woman is a great rarity, because it is the only case at our disposal with a *situs inversus and Kartagener's syndrome*, bearing in mind that only one in 32,000 people has this syndrome! Occasionally, luck is also on the side of doctors and physical anthropologists.[4]

## Notes

1. See chapter 9 above, on Greek cremations in Romania.

2. It is important to note that humans can have inversed organs without presenting with Kartagener's syndrome.

3. P. Charlier, G. Costea, I. Huynh-Charlier, L. Brun, G. Lorin de La Grandmaison, "Diagnosis of Aortic Dextroposition on Human Skeletal Remains," *Legal Medicine (Tokyo)*, 14/2, 2012, pp. 101–104.

4. See P. Charlier, G. Costea, A. Baralis, "Étude anthropologique et paléopathologique d'un sujet d'Aegyssus (III^e–IV^e siècle ap. J.-C., Roumanie)," *PEUCE* 7, 2009, pp. 337–346 and P. Charlier, G. Costea, I. Huynh-Charlier, L. Brun, G. Lorin de La Grandemaison, "Diagnosis of Aortic Dextroposition on Human Skeletal Remains," *Legal Medicine (Tokyo)*, 14/2, 2012, pp. 101–104.

# 16

## BAD CALCULUS

Urinary Calculus in a Roman Child
(2nd Century AD)

During the excavations of an imperial necropolis near Rome, osteoarchaeologist Paola Catalano exhumed the skeleton of a little six-year-old
girl who had lived in the 2nd century AD. Behind the pubic bone of this
skeleton, at the level of the bladder, there was a small, hard, crystalline
object, completely calcified, in the shape of a bean about one inch (2.5
cm) long. It corresponded to bladder stone lithiasis—in other words, the
stone or calculus is so large that it cannot be expelled through the natural
channels. This calculus was probably formed because of the hard water
that the young girl drank. Once formed in her bladder, this lithiasis could
have been the cause of chronic infections, but was not necessarily responsible for her death.

The interest of this discovery lay in its comparison with the recom-
mendations of Galen, a contemporary of the young girl, on evacuating
bladder stones in children, particularly little girls. To cure these lithiases,
Galen suggested drinking particular special waters which, according to
him, dissolved crystalline formations. In parallel, he recommended drinking other waters that allowed the size of the calculus to grow in order to
render them more fragile and thereby facilitate their evacuation. Finally,

in the worst cases, he suggested taking the child by the feet and shaking it, with the head down, in the hope that the calculus would fall. . . .

Had this young girl perhaps been treated by Galen? In any case, this discovery (and its interdisciplinary study) allows us to put the writings of an ancient doctor and a real anthropological case side by side.[1]

## Note

1. See P. Charlier, Y. Neuzillet, D. Fompeydie, W. Pantano, P. Catalano, C. Prêtre, J. Poupon, "Idiopathic Infantile Bladder Lithiasis from Roman Antiquity," *Urology* 78/1, 2011, pp. 1–2.

# 17

## NOT A WORD

### A Malformed Mouth in Roman Gaul
### (2nd Century AD)

At the time of the excavation and study of the Gallo-Roman necropolis of Lazenay, near Bourges, osteoarchaeologist Raphaël Durand (Inrap) had identified a serious malformation on the mouth of an adult male. He suffered from mandibular condylar aplasia—in other words, he was missing a part of the left extremity of his jaw that forms the junction with the base of the cranium (temporal) and that allows the opening and closing of the mouth. Clinically, our individual had a misaligned mouth with, in addition, an ankylosis that prevented him from opening it completely. Mandibular condyle aplasia is a birth defect, but it did not prevent this person from living a long time, since he died at around forty-five years of age. Though treatment was impossible for him at that time, he was nevertheless taken care of by the community, which most probably prepared a special diet for him.

This case illustrates that malformed individuals were not systematically eliminated at birth, as is often thought to be the case, and as is abundantly related in ancient texts. Even though that probability existed, archaeology proves that numerous malformed subjects were able to live in a social community without being excluded, and were sometimes taken care of by that society. However, there was probably a difference depending on the size of the settlement. In urban centers, belonging to an elite, or being close to it, or the religious beliefs of the time must have argued in favor of the elimination of a deformed being at birth; in the countryside, by contrast, one can reconstruct a radically different behavior. In the case that interests us here, the deformity of his jaw in no way prevented our patient from participating in agricultural work, and the community to which he belonged did not wish, or could not afford, to eliminate a potentially useful individual.[1]

## Note

1. See P. Charlier, R. Durand, I. Huynh, "Condyle Aplasia in an 1800-Year-Old Mandible from France," *Paleopathol Newsletter* 129, 2005, pp. 16–20.

# 18

## *RESQUIESCAT IN PACE*

A Lethal Trepanation and Another Successful One in
Imperial Rome (2nd Century AD)

The first case of interest to us is that of a cranium from the 2nd century AD, found in the necropolis of the Via Trionfale, in Rome, just next to the Vatican. In this necropolis there are both inhumations and cremations. Among the remains of one of them there was an oval bone fragment from the cranial vault, about the size of a spectacle lens. In spite of changes caused by exposure to fire, one can see that the entire circumference of this bone fragment is the result of a regular cut, apart from almost half an inch on one corner—it is a trepanation square. Our individual was trepanned during his lifetime, but the trepanation was not completed: the patient died during the surgical operation, probably as a result of a vascular lesion and massive bleeding. When the person died, the trepanation was abandoned, and the individual was incinerated, but this fragment of cranial vault escaped destruction. Rather paradoxically, this archaeological piece, which was a medical failure, allows us to reconstruct the therapeutic practices of ancient doctors. We do not know what this adult male patient was suffering from. Migraines? Headaches? A tumor? Infection? Trauma? No one will ever know. Had the entire skeleton come down to us, a more accurate diagnosis might have been possible.[1]

\*   \*   \*

The second case is a slightly happier one. It concerns the complete skeleton of a man who was more or less contemporaneous with the previous one, found in a necropolis in the southern suburbs of Rome (Via Villa di Settibagni, 1st to 3rd centuries AD). And this time we know why the person was trepanned: he had a fairly serious dental abscess that had spread septic metastases (collections of germs in the blood) that had grafted themselves onto a vertebra creating an abscess that opened secondarily toward the canal of the spinal cord. We do not know why the patient did not have his tooth pulled out, which would have allowed the pus to drain into the mouth, and probably would have avoided the spread of infection. Perhaps the patient belonged to some sort of aristocracy, and was concerned about his appearance. . . . But at that time, antibiotics did not exist. In any case, the infection went up into the cranium in the cerebrospinal fluid, and the patient was trepanned. Our man survived his trepanation, which was partly healed. But the inflammation continued in spite of everything, for the infection was still present on the inside of the cranial vault. The trepanation granted him a reprieve of a few weeks, it probably relieved the pain, but he ended up dying of that inflammation. This is a rare case because we know the precise medical reason for the trepanation, and because we have virtually the entire "medical file" on the patient.[2]

## Notes

1. See P. Charlier, L. Brun, W. Pantano, P. Catalano, I. Huynh-Charlier, "An Incomplete Fatal Trepanation Diagnosed on Cremation Remains" (Rome, Italy, 2nd c. AD). *Acta Medico-Historica Adriatica*, 2014, 12(2), pp. 315–320.

2. See P. Charlier, *Male mort. Morts violentes dans l'Antiquité*, Paris, Fayard, 2009, and P. Charlier, P. Catalano, S. Digiannantonio, "La paléochirurgie ou la naissance de la chirurgie. Une trépanation à Rome à l'époque impériale: un exemple pratique de neurochirurgie antique," *Journal de chirurgie*, 143/5, 2006, pp. 323–324.

# 19

## ATMOSPHERE, ATMOSPHERE . . .

A Child's Mummy from the Fin-Renard in Bourges
(2nd Century AD)

This is the story of the Gallo-Roman mummy of a child roughly three years old, found in Bourges in the 19th century in a stone sarcophagus inside which was a lead coffin containing said mummy in an excellent state of preservation. Only, not long after the discovery, children used the body of the mummy to play ball. . . . Contrary to what one might think today, and even if the behavior seems inconceivable to us, at the time this was not an isolated incident, and chronicles frequently mention this kind of spectacle. The most emblematic case is that of the Sorbonne: when the tomb of Richelieu was opened during the French Revolution, the people present played football with the cranium of the Great Cardinal. We do not know the reason behind this attitude: Was it perhaps a case of making fun of death, of playing with it, of warding off evil spirits?

Let us return to Bourges. The mummy was completely oxidized, which is logical: enclosed in a lead coffin for centuries, the entire body took on a color varying between brown and dark red. When a body decomposes in an airtight atmosphere such as this, there is an interaction with the metallic container, forming lead oxide which is deposited secondarily on the body in a gaseous or liquid form and acts as a fixative. The decomposition of the body then stops, and it dries out.

Doctor Thillaud coordinated the multidisciplinary study of this mummy. The numerous lesions (head detached from the body, arms torn out, various dislocations, etc.) were traumatic, but unburnished by time, attesting to blows received at the time of its discovery and thereafter. Examination under the microscope revealed that this child had red hair and that this was its natural color, not the result of oxidation of the lead coffin. It was not possible to establish the cause of death clearly, although tuberculosis seems the most likely. This child seems to have belonged to a local elite and benefited from a more prestigious burial that most of its contemporaries. Today, this little mummy is preserved in the Musée du Berry, in Bourges.[1]

## Note

1. See P.-L. Thillaud, Y. Glon, P. Charlier, J.-N. Vignal, "La momie du Fin-Renard (Bourges)," in D. Gourevitch, A. Moirin, N. Rouquet (eds), *Maternité et petite enfance dans l'Antiquité romaine*, Bourges, Service archéologique municipal, 2003, pp. 102–111.

# 20

# THE YELLOW PERIL

## "Fecal Peril" in Antiquity

It is a little-known fact that the main cause of mortality in antiquity was not war but the "fecal peril." Treatment of waste water was a real problem, and both the process of infection and the most basic rules of hygiene were completely unknown. At that time it was better to drink wine than water, at the risk of dying of cirrhosis at forty rather than of typhoid fever as an adolescent. . . . Even though some procedures for decontaminating water existed—vinegar was used, as is done today on a salad—they were often insufficient to prevent the absorption of germs.[1]

In paleopathology, we are interested not only in skeletons and texts, but also in artifacts that have a short period of contact with human beings. This brings us to a question that might seem trivial, but deserves to be asked: How did one wipe one's backside in Greco-Roman antiquity? A question that is all the more crucial because at that time, toilet paper did not exist; the oldest description of it in Western Europe dates back to the 16th century, whereas in China it had been used since the 2nd century AD. Over the centuries, techniques varied according to latitude and local customs of hygiene (e.g. animal fur, snow, seashells—and, failing everything else, the hand).

Let us return to Greco-Roman antiquity. The first possibility consisted of using a piece of one's toga; the second, of using large tree leaves; finally, of using a *tersorium*, a sort of sponge fixed on a stick firstly soaked in a basin of water, or in what one hoped was running water in the little channel passing below the latrines. In his *Letters to Lucilius*, Seneca tells of the death of a German gladiator who no longer wanted to fight and, having forced a *tersorium* down his throat, died of asphyxiation.

And then there were the *pessoï*, those little pieces of coarsely retouched pottery destined to wipe one's backside after defecation, which were used around all the Mediterranean under Roman domination. The diameter of these pottery pieces varied between an inch and a little over two inches (3 and 6 cm), and almost half an inch (1 cm) thick. Usually, any angles would have been removed in order to avoid any skin lesions (e.g. hemorrhoids, irritation of the mucous membrane, etc.) that developed through constant use—which occurred anyway, due to the abrasiveness of the pottery. The consequence of these lesions was even described by Horace in the 1st century BC. Regarding an elderly lady who had used these *pessoï* too much, he wrote: "You whose scrawny buttocks yawn with a hole more repugnant than the ass of a shitting cow." Once used, these *pessoï* were thrown in the latrines, or put in a receptacle, to be reused.

We also discovered that these *pessoï* could be used to vent: some had names engraved on them so that you wiped your backside with a *pessoï* bearing the name of your enemy. . . . In Athens and Piraeus, some have been found in latrines and in wells bearing famous names such as Themistocles, Pericles, and even Socrates.[2] For a long time, these were thought to be *ostraka*, the "slips" used for voting for or against the ostracism of an enemy, until it was discovered what other use they could be put to. . . .

\*　\*　\*

I had the opportunity of studying two *pessoï*, one from Crete and the other from Tunisia. These two artifacts came from old excavations of latrines, and on their surfaces there were still some deposits; by examining them under the microscope, I was able to detect remains of excrement and authenticate their use as sanitary items.

In Delos, during an "archaeological cleaning," I studied the latrines of a house located right in the theater quarter. The aim was to study and understand the waste water drainage system. The study, undertaken with archaeologist Yvon Lemoine, showed that the water conveyance coming from the upper floors, before it flowed down to the story below, was already full of excrement. This demonstrated the existence of latrines in the upper stories of houses, whereas previously it had been thought that they existed only at street level. Bones of small animals (mice, frogs) were also found in these latrines, which were attracted by this source of food. By contrast, and contrary to what we expected, there were no bones of children. During antiquity, the remains of miscarriages were, in fact, not infrequently thrown into latrines or, lacking a better option, into wells. There is a particularly interesting case in Ashkelon, Israel, where the latrines of a brothel contained the remains of 150 male newborns: the genetic study of these tiny skeletons showed that, in this establishment, baby girls were almost exclusively kept, to make prostitutes of them, while the boys were inevitably eliminated.

With a better understanding of the use of *pessoï* and of how latrines worked, and thanks to the study of contemporary texts, it is possible for us to learn a lot about daily life around the Mediterranean, about the hygiene of the time, and to build up a picture of sanitation in antiquity.[3]

## Note

1. On his way to the cross, Jesus was offered vinegar water. Contrary to popular belief, it was not a sign of contempt but rather a mark of deference: he was being offered the cleanest water available.

2. The reader should forgive me for this audacious parallel: the same procedure can be found today in Italy, where one can obtain toilet paper printed with the logo of Italian football clubs. It is thus possible for a supporter of Juventas, Milan, to wipe his backside with toilet paper representing AS Roma. . . .

3. See P. Charlier, L. Brun, C. Prêtre, I. Huynh-Charlier, "Toilet Hygiene in the Classical Era," *British Medical Journal*, 345, 2012, p. 8287.

# 21

## I AM ANOTHER . . .

An Embryonic Tumor in Rome (3rd Century AD)

We have already discussed the Roman necropolis of the Via Lucrezia Romana,[1] dating to the 2nd–3rd centuries AD, located next to a prestigious villa, and which mainly contained the skeletons of eastern slaves in the service of the residence. Among the skeletons of these slaves, there was one of a young woman (twenty-five to thirty-five years old), the study of which showed that behind the sternum there was a bony growth of about two to two and a quarter inches (5–6 cm), composed of poorly formed bone and containing some degraded teeth in its center.

This tumor is a teratoma; that is, according to the commonly accepted medical hypothesis, a twin that developed inside the body of this woman when she was in the amniotic sack. At a fairly early stage of her conception, her twin became stuck to her sternum, but it was destroyed by her body's immune system and its development was arrested, while that of the woman continued. Some teratomas can continue to develop, and in that case, the person finds him- or herself with a second body hanging on here and there. Teratomas are always found on the midline of the body, and they can produce two arm or two legs hanging from the thorax, but this does not prevent normal life. . . . We know of teratomas that have developed in the cranium, the palate, the nose, and the chin. Such cases have been known since antiquity; in 1530, Ambrose Paré made an accurate description of a case of a man about forty years old who lived in Paris, with his twin hanging from his belly.

These tumors may have been encouraged by the toxins that abounded in the Roman period. Contrary to what we believe currently, the state of health of the population at that time was far from impressive. During Roman antiquity, natural resources were intensively exploited, leading to pollution of the atmosphere, as well as the streams and rivers of entire regions. Jewelry was often made of contaminated metals, such as lead-bearing silver, and gold full of mercury or arsenic. Wearing this jewelry directly on the skin allowed the heavy metals to penetrate the body easily. Manganese was often present in the paint on vases or on pottery. Parasites such as malaria were a constant. And if one adds intestinal parasites and worms to this. . . . Taken altogether, these weaken the organism and produce a state of inflammation along with chronic immunodeficiency that can favor the occurrence of congenital malformations, or lead to death following only a modest infection. In this chrono-cultural context, most children at the time died in the week following their birth. Hence the tradition of not naming a baby before the seventh day. . . .

Regarding the case in question, our slave could live with this tumor with no problem, apart from slight breathlessness or a constriction of the chest, but the tumor was in no way responsible for her death. The teeth of the "twin" were degraded by the action of gastric or pancreatic juices. The fact that the teeth had deteriorated proves that the other embryonic tissues were present and that it was not simply a group of bones and teeth.

This type of discovery is exceptional: it was the first time that such a tumor had been discovered in physical anthropology.[2] Even though it is an isolated case, it allows us to say that teratomas have existed since antiquity and that this type of diagnosis can be made on a skeleton.[3]

## Notes

1. See Chapter 8, above, which discusses deformities.

2. Since then, another fairly similar case has been exhumed in Spain, also dating to the Roman period.

3. See P. Charlier, I. Huynh-Charlier, L. Brun, L. Devisme, P. Catalano, "Un tératome mature médiastinal vieux de 1800 ans," *Annales de pathologie* 29, 2009, pp. 67–69.

# III

## MIDDLE AGES

# 22

# PLAGUE OF . . .

A Hormonal Disease in Byzantine Crete
(7th Century AD)

This concerns a skeleton from the Byzantine site of Eleftherna, mentioned above, and excavated by Christina Tsigonaki. These skeletons are contemporary with the end of the Justinian plague in the 5th/6th centuries AD. So-called "catastrophe" graves were found there, containing four or five bodies per pit or sarcophagus. Currently, we do not know whether these grouped inhumations were due to the plague itself, to economic reasons, or, more prosaically, to a simple lack of space. Among these skeletons is one of a woman aged twenty-five to forty-five years, who has a very thick cranium, much thicker than normal, and the bones of her extremities are clearly hypertrophied. These initial "symptoms" already point to a diagnosis of acromegaly, in other words, an abnormal enlargement of the extremities—hands, feet, head—all clearly visible in the present case.

Acromegaly is an endocrine disease, linked to an over-secretion of the growth hormone by the pituitary gland. The pituitary fossa at the base of the cranium, which houses the pituitary gland, can be examined, and on this skeleton it is much too big, about three-quarters of an inch (2 cm) in diameter instead of the usual 8 mm. Most probably, this individual had a benign tumor around the pituitary gland, which gradually dilated the *sella turcica* and caused the inappropriate secretions of growth hormone, thereby producing the acromegaly. Acromegaly generates intracranial hypertension, which can be the cause of migraines and, more seriously, of brain hemorrhages. If the pressure of the pituitary gland becomes too great, the disease can become deadly by increasing the pressure on the carotids that pass just beside it. For this woman, the consequences also had a physical dimension: this disease produces a hypertrophied face, which renders the features more masculine.[1]

## Note

1. See P. Charlier, C. Tsigonaki, "A Case of Acromegaly (Greece, 7th Century AD)," *European Journal of Endocrinology*, 165/5, 2011, pp. 819–821.

# 23

# TWISTING THE NECK OF RECEIVED WISDOM

## A Congenital Stiff Neck in Byzantine Crete
## (7th Century AD)

This is the case of a patient from Argos, in Greece. The bones were brought to light in the 1950s by archaeologists from the French School in Athens and have been little studied since. Only two well-known anthropologists had taken a quick look.[1] The first, R. P. Charles, simply sexed the skeletons based on their crania, even though the pelvic bones were available.... A paleontologist by training, and an enthusiastic classifier, he was particularly interested by the "racial" distribution of Argive populations. The second, a certain J. L. Angel, anthropologist at the Smithsonian Institution in Washington, studied the crania that had been cleaned by Charles, with very personal preconceptions. In fact, he wanted to prove, at any cost, that malaria infested the region, and according to him, all the pathological lesions that he found attested to its presence. The storage conditions of these skeletons also dated from the 1950s, and rats feasted on the cardboard boxes that protected the bones. Nevertheless, this was a virtually unstudied collection of skeletons, covering a period stretching from the Mycenaeans to the Ottomans.

The first task was to rectify the determinations of sex that had been made, followed by a medical diagnosis of the bones. Over the course of this work, I found that it was possible to highlight a congenital stiff neck (torticollis) in one individual about forty years old, most probably a male.[2] The occipital hole, at the base of the cranium, which is normally a round or oval shape, was completely remodeled into a bean shape. This was the sign of a severe disease whose consequences for the patient were most probably serious from a neurological and orthopedic point of view. In general, this congenital disease is accompanied by anomalies in the spine (scoliosis) and a badly positioned neck and mouth.

However, despite this clearly visible malformation, the individual from the Byzantine period had been part of the community until an advanced age (at least forty years) and had not been disposed of at birth. This case shows us, yet again, that the preconceived notion of the systematic elimination of malformed babies in past populations is false. As such discoveries are made and diagnosed, osteoarchaeology can provide a different form of truth, one that is much more accurate than certain texts imply. Ancient texts perhaps indicate the path to follow, but not the path actually followed in daily life.[3]

### Notes

1. P. Charlier, "L'anthropologie grecque comme cheval de bataille: l'affrontement des écoles française et américaine dans l'étude des restes humains en Grèce" (1943–1985), *Eur. Rev. Hist.*, 2006, 4(13), pp. 643–660.

2. With the usual proviso, since only the cranium was preserved.

3. P. Charlier, I. Huynh, "Congenital Torticollis from Antiquity," *The Spine Journal*, 10/7, 2010, p. 655.

# 24

# THE AGE OF TARTAR

## Dental Tartar with Parasites

The reader little imagines what information we can find by examining the dental tartar of a human skeleton with a microscope. With a few exceptions, we can find *everything* that passed through the mouth of an individual. This method, developed about twenty years ago, has led to great advances in both forensics and archaeology. The teeth of every human being are covered by dental plaque that mainly contains saliva and includes numerous microscopic pieces of food residue. It is the gradual calcification of dental plaque that gives birth to tartar. When an individual dies, all this "information" remains fixed in the tartar, so that by analyzing it, we can understand his or her dietary habits better—and the corollary, dietary proscriptions—and we can also evaluate his or her state of health. Once a skeleton has been uncovered, and after extraction and decalcification of the tartar, it is possible, using a microscope, to identify food debris, even several centuries after the death of the patient. In this way we can find fragments of cereals, pollen, animal hairs, plants, parasites, even small insects that, trapped in the saliva, found themselves caught in irregularities of the teeth and were then covered with tartar. Using an electron microscope, it is possible to observe in yet greater detail, and to see bacteria, parasites, and even sperm.[1] Intestinal residues can also be found—for example, if an individual vomited a meal, parasites from the digestive system that come out through the mouth can become trapped in the dental plaque and then in the tartar. If an individual cleans his or her teeth, and this cleaning leads to bleeding, red blood cells can also find themselves trapped in the dental tartar and can inform us about the state of health of the patient. In this way, the study of Agnès Sorel's dental tartar showed traces of malaria, which was still rampant in France in the 15th century.

The study of dental tartar leads to advances in forensic medicine and provides information on the cause and circumstances of a death. Current research is concentrating on toxicological studies based on dental tartar, in order to find out whether an individual was poisoned by lead, arsenic, mercury, and so on, and also whether it is possible to identify any potential medical treatments.

The study of dental tartar also helps to solve some archaeological curiosities. Such is the case of an early 10th century AD skeleton found in Villiers-le-Bel, near Paris, buried in a disused grain silo, whose limbs had been cut off. Archaeologist Isabelle Abadie suspected that a specific pathology had been the cause of death of this individual and/or of his or her *post mortem* exclusion. Having studied the skeleton and found a fairly minor pathology, we sampled the dental tartar, of which there was quite a lot, on the individual's jaw. Its study revealed, for the first time in this chrono-cultural context, a parasite known as *Schistosoma haematobium*, an "exotic" parasite, responsible for urinary schistosomiasis, which exists only in Africa and Asia, not in Europe. What was this parasite doing in the Paris area? This individual's skeleton was found in a grain silo. As one might imagine, silos at that time bore no resemblance to contemporary silos. This was an "archaeological silo," dug into the ground, and it is not hard to believe that once no longer in use, it served as a grave—albeit an "atypical grave," different from that of the rest of the population.

The most likely conclusion to be drawn from this discovery is that the individual buried in the silo must have been either a traveler or a merchant, coming from Africa or Asia, who died in the Paris area. The fact that he was buried in an "atypical grave," or a "relegation grave," reinforces the idea that he was of no importance to the inhabitants of the place, and that they were satisfied with reusing a ready-made hole for his burial, rather than bothering to bury him with dignity, alongside the other inhabitants of the village. Unless he was carrying a really negative charge that represented a danger to the community of the living? Indeed, the bones were disarticulated *post mortem*: Did the inhabitants perhaps ward off fate by enacting a ritual of partitioning the corpse to avoid a scourge coming from elsewhere?[2]

## Notes

1. A sperm was found in the dental tartar of a young woman, about twenty-five years old, buried in an Italian necropolis of the 3rd century BC. Unfortunately, it is impossible to say whether this sperm was of the human or "food" type. In this particular case, the researcher was faced with two possibilities: either it was human sperm or it was the remains of food, from a dish containing "Rocky Mountain oysters"—in other words, lamb or bull testicles.

2. See P. Charlier, I. Huynh-Charlier, O. Munoz, M. Billard, L. Brun, G. Lorin de La Grandmaison, "The Microscopic (Optical and SEM) Examination of Dental Calculus Deposits (DCD): Potential Interest in Forensic Anthropology of a Bio-Archaeological Method," *Legal Medicine (Tokyo)*, 12/4, 2010, pp. 163–171, and P. Charlier, I. Abadie, S. Cavard, L. Brun, "Ancient Calculus Egg," *British Dental Journal*, 215/10, 2013, pp. 489–490.

# 25

# THE LORD OF ANJOU

The Tomb of Foulque Nerra III

The legendary Foulque Nerra III (972–1040), Count of Anjou, was a contemporary of Hugh Capet and his immediate successors and is considered to be the founder of the Plantagenet empire. He is particularly known for his spectacular U-turns, his excesses of all types, his warrior exploits, and his cruelty. And since our man was not short of a paradox or two, he was also renowned for his extreme religious devotion. Plunderer of monasteries, he was also a great builder of churches so that he might be pardoned. To this formidable warrior chief we owe the construction of numerous castles and strongholds. Foulque Nerra III, whose family was linked to the Pope, died at the very respectable age of sixty-eight years.

This man was also in the habit of disposing of his wives when he was bored with them, for political or matrimonial reasons. The most emblematic case is that of Elizabeth, who was accused of adultery—but the fact was that she had given him only a daughter—and who died in a fire while imprisoned in a church in Angers. Thanks to his skills and lack of scruples, the vast domain of Foulque Nerra III extended across much of the Val de Loire and was far more extensive than that of the king of France.

But such behavior when one is an important lord and close to the Pope can cause a few practical problems. To expiate his sins, Foulque Nerra undertook four pilgrimages to the Holy Land. During one of these journeys, he is said to have torn off a fragment of the Holy Sepulchre with his teeth,[1] brought it back to Beaulieu-lès-Loches, and had a basilica built, in which he wished to be buried. It still exists today.

In 1040, on returning from his fourth pilgrimage, Foulque Nerra III died in Metz, on the lands of his last wife. His body was opened and embalmed. The custom for pilgrims who died far from home was to cut the head and arms off so they could be displayed later. We do not know exactly what procedure was used on Foulque Nerra; the only thing we are sure of is that this is the oldest case of embalming for which there is a written record, the body having been prepared in Metz before being repatriated to the basilica at Beaulieu-lès-Loches, where it is said still to rest.

In 1869–1870, following a national archaeological congress at Loches, the archaeologists began an excavation project specifically to find the tomb of Foulque Nerra. A sarcophagus was removed from the place where the body was thought to be lying. A skeleton was found inside it and identified as being that of Foulque Nerra. The head was present and had not been sawed off; the forearms were still there, if somewhat degraded, and a few fragments of pottery and metal were also found. Once the excavation was finished, the sarcophagus was closed up and put back in its original place.

In 2007, with the authorization of the regional archaeological service, we undertook an "archaeological cleaning" of the tomb, followed by an anthropological study of the bones. The first observation was that the stone sarcophagus predated Foulque Nerra, which in itself is not illogical, for at the time it was the custom to rescue and reuse an older sarcophagus. However, the skeleton, which bore no arthritic lesions, was that of a man of about forty years—who had rickets on top of it all! The skeleton found in 1869–1870 did not correspond in any way with the historical descriptions of the person of the Count of Anjou: it must have been that of a canon or other member of the church who had been buried in the basilica.

This work showed that the body of Foulque Nerra III is probably still in Beaulieu-lès-Loches, but not where tradition places it. So where is it? It remains a mystery. The basilica has been heavily remodeled and maltreated over the years. Only further excavations might find the body of the terrifying Count of Anjou, and reveal how he was embalmed in 1040. A geophysical survey would be able to locate and examine the tomb. The most surprising thing in this story is that, over the years, houses were built on top of the basilica's ambulatory, which is the most likely place for him to have been buried. Without knowing it, people live several yards above the remains of the terrible Foulque, who is perhaps lying in their basement.[2]

## Notes

1. According to the account of his grandson, Foulque le Réchin, the count, having prostrated himself on the ground, his mouth on the earth, felt that a piece of the Sepulchre was detaching itself against his lips.

2. P. Charlier, A. Embs, Y. Ubelmann, M. Patou-Mathis, I. Huynh-Charlier, L. Lo Gerfo, "Le tombeau dit 'de Foulques Nerra III': étude archéologique et anthropologique," in P. Charlier (ed.), *Deuxième colloque international de pathographie (Loches, avril 2007)*, Paris, De Boccard, 2009, pp. 73–120.

# 26

## IN THE ODOR OF SANCTITY . . .

### The Heart of Richard the Lionheart

On April 6, 1199, having suffered in agony for about two weeks, Richard I, King of England, Duke of Aquitaine and Normandy, gave up his soul to God. Previously, on March 26, he had been seriously wounded in the shoulder by a crossbow bolt fired from the castle of Chalus, which he was besieging with his army. Poorly cared for, his wound rapidly degenerated into septicemia, and after several days of atrocious suffering, the sovereign expired, but not without having expressed his final wishes. As agreed, on the death of the king, a *dilaceratio corporis* was carried out; in other words, the king's body was separated into several anatomical entities. The political objective was to make a "marking" of territory after his death, by using these body fragments, which were of highly symbolic value. The heart was removed from the corpse, embalmed and put in a reliquary, which was itself placed under a stone effigy and deposited near the altar, in the choir of the cathedral of Rouen—the English capital in the so-called territory "of France." The body was embalmed and deposited in Fontevraud Abbey, in the Plantagenet cemetery, and rested under a magnificent polychrome effigy. And finally, a sign of the great Anglo-French friendship or a practical necessity commonly observed in examples of Medieval embalming, the entrails (the "lowest pieces" as it were) were left where they were. In other words, the intestines, lungs, and other organs of lesser importance were put in a casket for entrails, and deposited in the church of Chalus, the town in which he had died.

Richard the First of England rested in peace for several centuries, but during the Wars of Religion, the casket of entrails and its contents were sacked by the Protestants, as was the cemetery at Fontevraud. Of the late king of England, only the heart escaped the massacre, still preserved in Rouen.

The effigy of the heart of Richard the Lionheart was protected from the outrages of time in a fairly unusual fashion. A cathedral is, in fact, a permanent worksite. Over the centuries, the core of the building had been raised, and the effigy was completely buried under sediment and various masonry works undertaken during the subsequent raising of the choir. It had stayed in its original place in the cathedral, but, being invisible, it fell into oblivion.

Only in 1856 did a local antiquary find the effigy of the heart during renovation works on the building. Immediately next to the effigy, the reliquary was brought to light, intact. A small lead casket lined with silver, it had the following inscription on its lid: "Ici est le coeur de Richard, roi d'Angleterre" (Here is the heart of Richard, king of England). When it was "discovered," the reliquary was still sealed by the iron bars that closed it. The reliquary was opened at that time, and its contents tipped into another, crystal, reliquary. The original one is still in the cathedral treasury, but its contents were stored in the reserves of the departmental Museum of Antiquities in Rouen for fifty years, breaking (temporarily?) the wishes of the king to rest near the altar of the cathedral. . . .

Before any study of the reliquary, historical verifications on the identity of the subject were carried out. From this point of view, there was little or no doubt. All stages of the discovery of the reliquary were certified by witnesses and transcribed as official statements. The reliquary had not been desecrated at the moment of its discovery, in 1856. Witnesses at the time said that "the irons were intact." When we studied the new crystal reliquary, it had not been opened since the transfer in 1856. The initial scientific examination consisted in verifying that this was indeed a human heart, which was rapidly confirmed by a microscope study and the use of specific antibodies. Environmental pollens were also noted by Speranta

Popescu. By studying such pollen, a "pollen spectrum" can be established, through which the season of embalming can be dated and its location pinpointed with some precision. The results indicated the west-central region of France, in the months of March or April—which confirmed the historical documents that place the death of Richard the Lionheart at Chalus (Limousin) on April 6. Everything agreed: the viscera, the timing, and the geographic area.

Finding traces of frankincense was the first surprise. It is the oldest trace of frankincense found so far on western embalmed remains. Generally, we find spices and other embalming products, but not frankincense, which was rare and expensive. This detail is not trivial. In the Judeo-Christian tradition, frankincense smoke is used to establish a direct, and respectful, link between the chosen people and the divinity. In Exodus (30:34–38), Yahweh explains to Moses that the use of incense is strictly reserved for Him: "This incense shall be treated as most sacred by you. You may not make incense of a like mixture for yourselves; you must treat it as sacred to the LORD. Whoever makes an incense like this for his own enjoyment of its fragrance, shall be cut off from his people." Later, incense reappears at the very beginning of the life of Jesus, when it was brought by the magi, along with myrrh and aloes. If the heart of Richard the Lionheart was embalmed in incense, it was no coincidence: when King Richard died, he had a few faults that needed forgiving—dubious sexuality, abuses during the Third Crusade, and so on. Shortly after the death of the king, the Bishop of Rochester declared that the deceased would expiate his crimes in purgatory for thirty-three years—a symbolic number—before being able to go to paradise. Using incense to embalm Richard's heart was intended to reduce the waiting time. The study of King Richard's heart also revealed other embalming products, such as rose, mint, myrtle, lime, and even a piece of mercury. These many plants served to give the heart a very special smell, the infamous "odor of sanctity," but this one was artificial.

Unfortunately, it was not possible to undertake Carbon-14 dating nor to extract DNA from the king's heart. To obtain these, it would have been necessary to destroy almost all the remains of the heart, and without any guarantee of a reliable result. This technical problem makes any analysis that would deprive future generations of the study material ethically delicate. But it is not beyond the realm of possibility that in the near future, new technologies will be able to analyze these remains while destroying only an infinitesimal portion. Frustration was all the greater because at the time these analyses were being undertaken, archaeologists in Leicester, England, had found the skeleton of Richard III, the Lionheart's distant descendant, under a parking lot. A comparative study of the DNA could have confirmed or refuted the kinship between the two kings, were there any doubt.

It seems incredible to some historians and chroniclers that Richard the Lionheart died in such a "stupid" and "simple" way. Conspiracy theorists very quickly put together some fairly audacious hypotheses. According to the heralds of the English king, the fatal crossbow bolt was poisoned. Another plot put forward was that the doctors did everything to cause the sovereign's death by taking poor care him. We would object firstly that the death of Richard the Lionheart is very "logical." A death on the battlefield—or during a siege in this case—was one of the risks of the trade. An aggravating circumstance was that when the king of England was hit by the crossbow bolt, he was not wearing chain mail. Although analysis of the heart of King Richard revealed many bacteria and fungi, we do not know if these were linked to the cause of death (septicemia) or to the decomposition or putrefaction process of the organ. In any case, no trace of poisoning (arsenic, for example) was found.[1]

## Note

1. P. Charlier, J. Poupon, G. F. Jeannel, D. Favier, S. M. Popescu, R. Weil, C. Moulherat, I. Huynh-Charlier, C. Dorion-Peyronnet, A. M. Lazar, C. Hervé, "The Embalmed Heart of Richard the Lionheart (1199 A.D.): A Biological and Anthropological Analysis," *Scientific Reports*, 3, 2013, pp. 1296 ff.

# 27

# ALL ROTTEN!

## The Charnel Houses for Medieval Bodies

The small church of Sainte-Mesme, in Yvelines, conceals a little-known treasure, a medieval charnel house. It was discovered by a local amateur archaeological society in a crypt, unknown until then, under the village church, and it contained some human bones. The town hall contacted a team of experts, who gathered to examine this unusual discovery.

The charnel house of Sainte-Mesme is a crypt located under the choir of the medieval building, as close as possible to the altar concealing the sacred relics. It is reached by descending an access staircase composed of seven steps. At the bottom are two parallel pits ten feet (3 m) long and about four-and-a-half feet (1.4 m) deep, separated by a low wall of white-washed rubble. Following the death of an individual, the body, wrapped in its shroud, was laid on wooden (or metal) bars and slowly decomposed. The bodily fluids dripped into the pit and amalgamated with the earth. When the body had "returned to dust," only the completely defleshed cranium and long bones, such as the femur, tibia, humerus, etc., remained, for they could not fall through the wooden bars. About a year after death, the bones were retrieved and they were put into an ossuary located either in a chapel or in a place reserved for this purpose in the cemetery. This funerary practice, onerous in terms of both time and money, was reserved exclusively for the local nobility. The aim of this rite was that the body should decompose as close as possible to the saint (*ad sanctos*), in order to benefit from that proximity. During the transformation of the body, the saint could thus intercede for the soul of the deceased to enter paradise rapidly, with the shortest possible time in purgatory.

It is quite rare to be able to examine a medieval charnel house in good condition, with its architecture intact. The charnel house of Sainte-Mesme was in use until the early 16th century, when the bars were removed and the large pits reused to hold bodies. Skeletons of an adult and of a child from the 16th century were found there.

The cranium of that child showed clear traces of cutting, with complete sawing of the skull cap and residues of embalming products. Graffiti dating to the late 18th century were discovered, which prove that the site had been visited by "tourists" of a particular type—like many other aristocratic tombs, those located in the charnel house of Sainte-Mesme were looted during the French Revolution. Officially, the revolutionaries opened the graves to salvage the lead of the sarcophagi and melted it down to make "patriotic bullets." More prosaically, they stole the gold found on the remains and sullied the memory of those dead who had oppressed them. . . . The vault of Sainte-Mesme was desecrated at that period. The bodies had been left where they were, but much disturbed. Small bones were also found in the charnel house. These were probably bones that had fallen between the wooden struts and that had not been retrieved and placed in the ossuaries. Some objects were still present, such as shroud pins, the use of which goes back to the Middle Ages.

This scientific study allowed us to learn more about the organization of charnel houses and how they functioned. The good state of preservation also meant that its history could be reconstructed, from its creation in the Middle Ages until it was looted in the 18th century. Clearly, its original use evolved, but it was always reserved for the local aristocracy. A genetic test could have determined whether the bones belonged to the same family or clan. Nowadays the charnel house of Sainte-Mesme is closed and cannot be visited because it is too cramped. But anyone visiting the church of Sainte-Mesme will be able to see a small slab near the altar, which is its door. The visitor will understand why incense is used during liturgical ceremonies: in this case, the mustiness rising from the crypt was probably not always the odor of sanctity. . . . [1]

## Note

1. P. Charlier, Y. Ubelmann, I. Huynh-Charlier, J. Poupon, "Les pourrissoirs médiévaux de l'église paroissiale Sainte-Mesme (Yvelines): étude architecturale et ostéo-archéologique," in P. Charlier (ed.), *Deuxième colloque international de pathographie*, op. cit., pp. 211–232.

# 28

# AN ANATOMY LESSON

The Oldest Anatomical Dissection (13th Century)

Here is an anatomical piece worthy of the greatest museums, yet it is part of a private collection, in Anvers, Belgium. Bought on the art market in the 1950s or '60s—such a sale would be impossible today[1]—this ancient human torso, from the pectorals to the cranium, is the oldest known anatomical dissection in the world.

When the collector acquired this unique piece, it had been sold to him as being one of the four torture victims supplied to André Vésale and Ambroise Paré at the death of Henri II. Let us look at the legend. According to a story completely fabricated in the 19th century, worthy of a novel by Alexandre Dumas, when Henri II found himself seriously injured in the right eye after his fatal tournament, as he lay dying, Catherine de Medici summoned some famous practitioners to his bedside: André Vésale and Ambroise Paré. The queen is also said to have given each of them two men condemned to death at the Châtelet, impaled in the face in the same way as the king. The man of science who managed to save one of these guinea pigs would then have been in charge of looking after the king. The whole story is pure invention.

A quick morphological and anatomical examination of the torso sweeps away this pretty legend, constructed solely around an opening in one eye. Deeper examination (Carbon-14 dating, medical scan, genetic analysis, etc.) shows us that this male body dates to the 13th century AD and that it is unique. In fact, at the moment of death, or a few minutes after this person died, mercury mixed with bees wax and olive oil was injected into the aorta, just where it leaves the heart. The intention had been to fill the arteries, to make them red and visible from the exterior (something like an arteriogram or angiogram today), to fix the tissues (mercury is good for preserving, like formaldehyde), and thereby to preserve the anatomical piece. Over the years, this piece was used for anatomical explorations. The brain was extracted, the dura mater was preserved, the left eye and the thyroid gland were explored by the practitioner. The piece smells very good, for it was smoked, either to help preserve it or to repel woodworm that had started to infest it.

We tried to find out which practitioner might have been responsible for such an anatomical piece in the 13th century. Our most likely "suspect" would be Guillaume de Salicet (1210–1277), practicing in Padua at that time, who had easy access to cadavers and who was particularly interested in these areas of anatomy. Such preparation must have helped him in his medical practice, or even for teaching—unless it was part of a "cabinet of curiosities" of the time.

Contrary to what is thought today, in the Middle Ages there was no prohibition by the Catholic Church concerning dissections, and even less against autopsies with a forensic view aimed at shedding light on suspicious deaths. There simply existed a regulation to prevent looting and misbehavior in cemeteries by medical students, for it was not unusual to see fresh graves regularly defiled. From the Middle Ages to the 19th century, those close to the deceased stayed near the cemetery for the week following death to keep watch over the dead until the body putrefied—and became unusable to medical students. This makes this anatomical piece all the more precious. Perhaps one day it will join the collections of a museum to be exhibited to the general public—if such is its place.[2]

### Notes

1. Since the so-called "Huriet" law on bioethics of 1994.
2. See P. Charlier, I. Huynh-Charlier, J. Poupon, E. Lancelot, P. F. Campos, D.

Favier, G. F. Jeannel, M. Rippa Bonati, G. Lorin de La Grandmaison, C. Hervé, "A Glimpse into the Early Origins of Medieval Anatomy Through the Oldest Conserved Human Dissection (Western Europe, 13th c. A.D.)," *Archives of Medical Sciences*, 10/2, 2014, pp. 366–373.

# 29

# THE MAGIC MOUNTAIN

## Human Diseases in the Greek Orthodox
## Art of Mount Athos

While waiting for the results of the competitive examination for a medical internship, I had been given authorization by His All Holiness Bartholomew, Ecumenical Patriarch of Constantinople, for an extended stay on Mount Athos, under the aegis of the French Society for the History of Medicine.

It is worth describing the arrival at this magical place, far away from everything. When a traveler passes over the threshold of the monastery of Mount Athos, whoever he is, as a sign of hospitality he is offered a glass of water, a glass of raki, and a rose-flavored Turkish delight. Next, the monks ask: "Where are you from? Why have you come? What can we do for you?" In reply, I gave my *diamonitron*, my safe-conduct, which comes in the form of a parchment, signed by Bartholomew with a sort of bulla, which allowed me to stay there more than two days. But in exchange for hospitality, the visitor must participate in at least one religious service per day and must be of service to the community—washing dishes, sweeping, or, for the young doctor that I was, examining the small pathologies (sometimes intimate) of the monks.

The first part of my work consisted in examining the medical libraries of several Greek monasteries in order to establish the provenance of the works: Amsterdam, Venice, Constantinople, Seville, Paris, etc. Mapping of the origins of the medical books was done, as well as mapping of pharmacy and botany. The second stage comprised the study of representations of diseases on the frescoes showing the miracles of Christ, such as the healing of the blind, of the paralytic, and of the man with an edema. The point was to see how diseases were reproduced, to recognize in them the influence of medical treatises and of particular painters. Most of the frescoes at Mount Athos were made by the Cretan school between the 14th and 16th centuries, a period that corresponds with the Byzantine Renaissance and its continuation, following the fall of Constantinople. That school had its origins on the Mediterranean island of Crete which, occupied by the Venetians at the time, found itself at the crossroads of Italian, Oriental, and Greek Orthodox influences. Its style is Byzantine neo-figurative, but with more modern techniques and diverse influences. At Mount Athos, one of the frescoes is inspired directly by Dürer's *Four Horsemen of the Apocalypse*. It was made just fifteen years or so after the publication of the woodcut. Among the most important artists of the 16th century who worked at Mount Athos, one should mention Theophanes the Cretan and his son Simeon, who decorated numerous orthodox monasteries. Fresco artists continued to work until the 18th century, after which all went still.

The diversity of sources and influences in a place that is rather difficult to access and is isolated from the world is striking. Such variety of origins can be explained by journeys the monks made to other monasteries, to Constantinople, or during missions, pilgrimages, councils, etc., and by the significant circulation of books. Finally, the fresco artists themselves traveled a lot and were inspired by artistic movements in the countries they crossed, notably by Flemish and German painting.

Often, anatomic realism suffered. Although some pathologies were represented well, such as an edema, this was not the case for numerous other diseases, notably skin diseases and paralyses, which were idealized rather than represented.[1]

## Note

1. See P. Charlier, "Iconographie des maladies humaines dans l'art grec ortho-doxe: l'exemple du mont Athos," *Histoire des sciences médicales*, 1/37, 2003, pp. 105–122.

# 30

# WITH A VALIANT HEART . . .

## The Mummy of Saint Rose

Born to a poor family in 1235 in Viterbo, Saint Rose passed most of her short life in contemplation and penitence. She died March 6, 1252, still in Viterbo, and was canonized in 1457 by Pope Callixtus III. When she died, her body was deposited in the town's convent and, six months later, it was still intact. Her grave then became a place of pilgrimage around which many miracles occurred.

Recently, a team of Italian experts was granted permission to carry out a detailed examination of the body. The mummy was still in good condition. Initial studies showed that this was indeed the body of a woman aged about twenty. But this anthropological examination of the mummy of Saint Rose of Viterbo was not without surprises. In fact, when they examined the inside of the body with a fiberscope, they noticed that the torso had no sternum! This is a known medical pathology: Saint Rose of Viterbo suffered from agenesis of the sternum, the ribs were joined to each other by cartilage and not by the usual bone. During life, when pressure was applied to her chest, it all sank into her body.

The other peculiarity of this mummy was revealed by the study of the heart, which had been separated from the body and placed in a reliquary, but had not been embalmed. Following an external examination then a scan of the heart, the team deduced that she had a dilated ventricle, and that she died of thrombosis. The discovery was published at the time in the prestigious medical journal *The Lancet*.

But having read the article, and having looked at the images with a forensic eye, I suggested that the thrombus of Saint Rose could have occurred *post mortem*: at the moment when the heart had been removed from the body, blood could very easily have coagulated inside the ventricle. Only microscopy could determine whether the blood had clotted while the individual was alive, or whether it had clotted *post mortem*.

Examination with the naked eye and with a scanner does not always allow an accurate diagnosis: an image is an invaluable tool, but its interpretation can be subject to controversy. When possible, the diagnosis should be confirmed or invalidated categorically by more in-depth studies. Thus, in addition to the methods used previously, microscopy can also provide answers. In the case of the heart of Saint Rose of Viterbo, for reasons of preservation of the relic, a re-examination had not been foreseen (it would have required opening the heart to take a sample). But, in the near or distant future, it might be possible to undertake such a study and finally provide an accurate medical answer regarding the causes of her death.[1]

## Note

1. See P. Charlier, "No Proof that Santa Rosa Heart Thrombus was Antemortem," *Lancet*, 376/9746, 2010, p. 1052.

# 31

# A VASE IN THE CRANIUM

## The Reliquary of Saint Afra (13th Century)

This reliquary comes from a private collection in Barcelona, and we undertook an interdisciplinary study of it. According to Catholic tradition, Saint Afra had lived in Augsburg, Bavaria, in the 3rd century AD. Of Cypriot origin, she was destined to become a priestess of Venus. Following the death of her husband, the king of Cyprus, Afra's mother left the island with her daughter and took refuge in Augsburg. Thereafter, all we know about the life of Saint Afra is that she lived the life of a prostitute (some sources mention that she ran a brothel)[1] and that in one night she was converted to Christianity by Bishop Narcissus, who had taken refuge in her establishment and whom she was protecting from anti-Christian persecution. Arrested the following day, she refused to sacrifice to the pagan gods and declared to her executioners: "My sins are numerous enough for me not to add this one. My martyrdom will serve as my baptism." Led to her torture, some sources say that she was burned, others recount that she was attached to a tree and decapitated along with her mother, Saint Hilaria of Augsburg, and three of her servant girls. Afra was recognized as a saint by the Catholic Church in 1064, and her feast day is August 5. We do not know how her reliquary could have arrived in this private collection.

The reliquary consists of the top of a cranium, silver-plated, tucked away inside an oak box lined with red velvet. A hole a few inches wide had been made in the silver reliquary so that the faithful could see or touch the relic and bless shreds of cloth. The organization of the relic itself dates to the 15th century. It consists of a piece of green silk about eight inches (20 cm) long, entirely sewn up, closed by three symbolic golden seals and still bearing an *authentication*, in other words an inscription on parchment bearing witness to the authenticity of the relics. This one for Saint Afra was written in cursive Castillian and was easy to read: "*[hoc est] caput sanctae virginis nobilis de societate undecim millium virginum* ([This is the] cranium of Saint Afra, virgin of noble family, one of the eleven thousand virgins)."[2] It seems that the relic had not been disturbed since the 15th century. The owner of this relic wanted to know if it really was of human origin, because the cranium seemed small to him, and inside, everything seemed fragmented. Since cutting the cloth surrounding the relic was out of the question, we made a scan.

The results confirmed that it was a human cranium that presented numerous fractures due to careless handling. Despite its poor condition, the cranium presented a majority of female characteristics, but only a deeper study of other parts of the body would allow us to be certain. A microscopic sample of dental tartar was taken from a tooth found separately in the reliquary. It did not show any particular anomalies. Although the lower part of the body was missing, there was no evidence of decapitation. The cranial vault had been fractured by much handling and the bones were sometimes superimposed in three or four layers, which would explain the "fragmented" feel of the cranium when it was touched. The inside of the cranium was filled with stuffing, but the most surprising part of this examination is that it revealed the presence of a small flagon in the cranium of the relic. One and a half inches (4 cm) high, it had been placed by the occipital bone. No stopper was visible, but it seemed to contain something. X-ray densities suggested that this vase was not of metal, but rather of ceramic or glass. What was it doing in the cranium of Saint Afra?

Through an old and small tear in the cloth, a supple fiberscope explored the relic and provided many answers to our questions. The stuffing was cotton, with a few strands of plants; the vase, of blown glass, contained bone dust and was closed at the neck by an authentication of paper that mentioned the name of Saint Claudian. Just next to it, another, coarser manuscript bore the inventory of the various saints whose remains had been grouped with Afra's cranium: Claudian, Victoire, and Phillip. Thus, we were in the presence of the only known case of a relic reliquary!

To date the relics, we compared the writing on the authentications. That of Saint Afra dates to the late 14th or early 15th century: the style of writing was current in Spain in the early 15th century. The writing on the authentication of Saint Claudian is that of a clerk from the second half of the 16th century, and the very fine paper was typical in Spain at the time. The third authentication, more difficult to decipher, mentions the "dust" (ashes) of Saint Claudian, Saints Phillip and Anaclet, Saint Victoria, Saint Sebastian, Saint Sabina, "and other martyrs" from the Spanish towns of Villalonga, near Valencia, and Benidorm, from where these fragments or relics must have come.

In conclusion, we can say that we are in the presence of a young adult female cranium which, since the 15th century, has been presumed to be that of Saint Afra, except that the cranium shows no trace of decapitation or cremation, and that it was damaged long ago by much handling. The relic must have come from Villalonga. A restructuring was carried out in the 17th or 18th centuries, with the addition of other relics: those of Saint Claudian, which are still there, and relics of other martyrs, which seem to have disappeared—only their authentication remaining inside the cranium.

But are these really the relics of Saint Afra? Unfortunately, it is impossible to answer categorically. If we base things on the story carried down by Catholic tradition, the reply is no, because the relic shows no traces of the presumed martyrdom. However, its authentication refers to the "eleven thousand virgins" massacred by the Huns in 383, near Cologne. This legend, which appeared in the 10th century, was popularized between 1261 and 1266 by Jacques de Voragine in the *Golden Legend*, but relies on highly controversial historical facts. Indeed, the author does not mention the name of Saint Afra among the eleven thousand virgins. On the other hand, he evokes the name of Saint Victoria, daughter of Saint Ursula, who died in similar circumstances. The mystery thus remains complete.

An interesting detail: other relics of Saint Afra exist in Germany. Indeed, the St.-Afra-in-the-Fields Church in Friedeberg, near Augsburg, was built on the very spot where, according to tradition, she had been executed. In addition, a Late Roman sarcophagus in the ancient basilica of Saint Ulrich and Saint Afra in Augsburg is presented as being that of Saint Afra, a relic of whom is preserved in the church of Saint John of Ebringen-in-Hegau. Will further research perhaps pierce this mystery one day?[3]

## Notes

1. Thus Saint Afra is invoked, among others, by repentant prostitutes.

2. This authentication therefore refers to an Afra who was one of the eleven thousand sacrificed virgins, whose story is told in the *Golden Legend*.

3. P. Charlier, I. Huynh, P.-L. Thillaud, F. Pannier, F. Reynaud, J.-L. Lemaître, "Étude pluridisciplinaire du reliquaire de sainte Afra (Barcelone)," in P. Charlier (ed.), *Premier colloque international de pathographie (Loches, avril 2005)*, Paris, De Boccard, 2006, pp. 59–70.

# 32

# TRAFFICKING IN RELIQUARIES

The Fake Reliquaries of Joan of Arc (15th Century)

At the time when I was working on the remains of Agnès Sorel, I went to the museum of the Amis du vieux Chinon (Friends of Old Chinon) to make an inventory of strands of hair of the so-called "dame de Beauté" (see the following chapter), one of which was held in this establishment. In the museum's reserves, just next to this strand of hair, was a reliquary known by the name of "bottle of Chinon," containing bones that looked carbonized and with a label reading: "Remains said to be of Joan of Arc." This type of relic was undeniably of anthropological and forensic interest. We know that after Joan of Arc was burned alive, her remains were thrown into the River Seine in order to prevent "acts of sorcery seeing the light of day based on her relics."[1] The text accompanying the "bottle of Chinon" was, moreover, cautious regarding the relics' authenticity. A few years later, I returned to Chinon armed with the joint authorization of the Archbishop of Tours and the Association des Amis du Vieux Chinon to carry out a scientific analysis of the remains.

The death of Joan of Arc is the best-documented execution of the 15th century. Thanks to her retrial and the abundance of testimonies gathered on that occasion, we know the circumstances precisely of her death, which occurred on May 30, 1431, on the Place du Vieux-Marché in Rouen.

As a general rule, when an individual is burned alive—a classic punishment in the Middle Ages—the pyre was lit and the victim, sewn into a sack, was thrown into the furnace. Combustion was rapid, as was death, which occurred within minutes. If need be, the executioner could shorten the agony with a pike. . . . For Joan of Arc, the English used a different, much lengthier, procedure, one that did not hide the victim from the eyes of the crowd. The English were determined that the people should see her die so that "no-one could claim that she had escaped or that another woman had been substituted in her place."[2]

The execution was carried out in three stages. Poisoned by the vapors, Joan of Arc died while only her dress had been burned by the flames. Appearing dead and naked to the crowd, straw was added near the body and the inferno was revived. Next, the bindings that held Joan came loose and the body fell into the inferno. After a fairly long time, the executioner ascertained that the heart and entrails of Joan of Arc were not burnt (which would be considered a miracle during the canonization trial) and piled charcoal, oil, and sulfur on the said organs to hasten their combustion. Finally, the ashes of the maiden of Orleans were collected and thrown into the Seine. If one believes the inscription on the lid of the "bottle of Chinon," an individual must have collected the remains of Joan of Arc that fell *under* the masonry platform that held the pyre.

No one hears anything about these supposed relics until 1867, when the remains of Joan of Arc are "discovered" in the attic of a pharmacy, in the Rue du Temple in Paris, that was due for demolition by the works of Baron Haussmann. Its proprietor, who knew nothing of the existence of this relic, gives it as a gift to Sylvain Noblet, a student of pharmacy, who, without opening it, along with Ernest-Henry Tourlet and his pharmaceutical student friends, identifies the contents. The cap of the bottle carried this inscription: "Remains found/under the pyre of Joan of Arc/maiden of Orleans." The writing is a cursive script from the 17th or 18th centuries. In 1867, Noblet gives the bottle to his friend Ernest-Henry Tourlet, who then moved to Chinon. Up to now, the bottle has still not been opened. In 1891, Tourlet gets in touch with the commission set up in Orleans to study Joan of Arc's cause with a view to her canonization. He authorizes that commission to make an opening in the bottle to study the relics, on condition that its members are irreproachably serious. On October 25, 1892, the bottle arrives, but it has been fractured by the bumpy journey. A hole two inches by three-quarters of an inch (5 × 2 cm) thus exists, allowing the contents to be removed without touching the parchment of the cap. The commission gathers on October 28 and December 15, 1892. It is presided over by the Bishop of Orleans and constituted of two doctors from the Hôtel-Dieu, one pharmacist-chemist, one paleography expert, a photographer, and several ecclesiastics. In 1893, Canon Desnoyers, director of the Musée Historique et Archéologique de l'Orléanais, writes a general report concluding that the fragments of bones included "a human false rib charred by fire and covered by a thick blackish coating of balm in which pitch or one of its derivatives dominates." Also identified are an envelope of coarse hemp cloth from the 15th century and two pieces of oak. Curiously enough, this report remained unpublished until 1972. On October 18, 1909, a new episcopal commission gathers in house of the the widow Tourlet, who is now the owner of the relic, and the remains are transferred into two new cylindrical bottles, which were sealed. In 1938, the widow Tourlet gives these remains to Abbot Gentet, curate of Saint Maurice of Chinon. In 1956, the two bottles are lent to Régine Pernoud for the exhibition *Jeanne d'Arc et son temps* (Joan of Arc and her times) in Rouen and Paris, to celebrate the 500th anniversary of her rehabilitation trial. In 1963, the bottles and their accompanying documents are given over to André Boucher, president of the Amis du Vieux Chinon. In 1974, the remains are once again transferred. In 1979, a fragment of wood is sent to Dr. W. G. Mook at the University of Groningen in the Netherlands, who concludes that it dates to 1700/1900 BC. On January 5, 1983, the remains are grouped together in a cardboard box and placed in the museum's stores. Thanks to these documents, we have fairly accurate evidence of the travels of these famous relics, from their "discovery" in the mid-19th century until today. And, as one might suspect given the dating of the piece of wood, there is some reservation regarding their authenticity.

With a multidisciplinary team and the most modern forensic techniques, we have studied these relics. It quickly became clear that they were the remains of several Egyptian mummies, which had not been burnt (no trace of carbonization was found) but were covered with a blackish balm (bitumen and pitch) which, from a distance, could give the illusion of a cremation. The cloth, a very good quality linen, was equally compatible with material from the 15th century as with pharaonic fabric. Some of the pollen examined belonged to unspecified members of the pine family. In addition, one of the bones in the reliquary was from a cat, which had also not been burned, and which was of a Near Eastern, not a European, species. Finally, the Carbon-14 dating placed these bones between the 7th and 3rd centuries BC. The relics of Joan of Arc were in fact remains of Egyptian mummies from the late period. The "burnt" aspect of the bones was due to the embalming products used at that time. In addition to these studies, Robert Montagut (national expert in apothecary jars and objects of curiosity) examined the manuscript inscription on the bottle of Chinon. The results of his analysis argue in favor of a fake, written in the 19th century but in an archaic fashion, imitating an older style (17th or 18th centuries).

*  *  *

Henceforth, it was clear that we were dealing with false relics, made to order, with a pseudo-history of discovery in an attic to increase their authenticity. But who was responsible for this fake? Noblet? Tourlet? Was it a hoax? A joke by a medical student that was taken seriously? We do not know. However, the origin of the bones points us toward a member of the medical corps. Indeed, the remains of mummies (the *mummia*) had been used in pharmacopoeia since the 15th century. It was easy for a pharmacist to make such a relic, but the deception still had to work.

The other interesting aspect of this story is the date at which the relic appears: 1867. Contrary to what is often thought, the memory of Joan of Arc did not endure after her death and she fell into oblivion until her rediscovery, in the mid-18th century, when she once again became a popular figure (a heroine of the common people who saved the kingdom), notably in stories by Voltaire. When the relic appeared, in 1867, the Maid of Orleans became the subject of a fierce and iconic battle among communists, socialists, nationalists, and Christians. Were these false relics made to create a palpable substratum of the Maid of Orleans for the faithful and thereby ensure the victory of one camp over the other? The question can be raised.

In any case, these remains have led to the establishment of an interdisciplinary scientific protocol for the study of fragmented remains that look burnt. It is a useful protocol for solving forensic cases, and participating in the "demonstration of truth."[3]

## Notes

1. Cochard, "Existe-t-il des reliques de Jeanne d'Arc ?," *Mémoires de la société archéologique de l'Orléanais*, 23, 1891, 191 p. (and an additional memoir of 23 pages dated to 1900).

2. *Ibid.*

3. See P. Charlier, J. Poupon, A. Eb, P. de Mazancourt, T. Gilbert, I. Huynh-Charlier, Y. Loublier, A.-M. Verhille, C. Moulheirat, M. Patou-Mathis, L. Robbiola, R. Montagut, F. Masson, A. Etcheberry, L. Brun, E. Willerslev, G. Lorin de La Grandmaison, M. Durigon, "The 'Relics of Joan of Arc': A Forensic Multidisciplinary Analysis," *Forensic Science International*, 194/1–3, 2010, pp. 9–15.

# 33

# THE "DAME DE BEAUTÉ"

Agnès Sorel (c. 1422–1450)

On February 7, 1450, Agnès Sorel arrived at the manor of Vigne, in Mesnil-sous-Jumièges. Barely had she settled in when she was suddenly afflicted with a "stomach flux" (dysentery) and died two days later (February 9) at six pm, with a loud cry, but not without having previously commended her soul to God and made considerable grants to the Saint Ours of Loches collegiate church, where she wished to be buried. The "beautiful Agnès" was then aged 28 and had just given birth to a stillborn premature baby of seven months. Very soon, suspicions would grow regarding the cause of death of the favorite of Charles VII. Assassination? Poisoning? Suicide? Who could have held a grudge against the "Dame de Beauté," as she was known then? According to her wishes, Agnès Sorel was interred in the choir of the church, and a magnificent funerary monument was erected there. Her body was embalmed, her heart removed and buried in the Abbey of Jumièges but, contrary to tradition, her cranium was not sawed.

Soon after, the canons began asking the successive kings if they would kindly move the effigy, not only because it obstructed the religious offices but also because the "bad morals" of the lady did not justify such a choice position in a sacred place. . . . Louis XI, who had often opposed his father's mistress, agreed that the body could be exhumed, on the sole condition that the canons return the gold that she had had given to them when she was alive. The cupidity of the canons cancelled the transfer. . . . It was only in 1777 that the clerics finally succeeded in convincing Louis XVI that this effigy obstructed the religious offices and that they obtained the long-awaited exhumation. On March 5, 1777, the effigy was moved, the tomb opened and the three coffins (two of wood and one of lead) broken. The remains of Agnès Sorel were then collected with care, placed in a sand-stone pot, and the whole (effigy and remains) transferred to elsewhere in the nave. In spite of the proscription against taking parts of the body, a braid of hair was cut off and divided among several people. An official report and two testimonials related the conditions of this exhumation in detail, which seems to have been more like the moving of bones to make space for additional bodies.

In 1793, the grave was defiled by the revolutionaries who believed they were linked to a saint. One Coulaine, witness to this defilement, related in a letter:

> I entered by chance into the collegiate church where there were several curious onlookers busy watching the demolition of the marble mauso-leum of Agnès. From below this mausoleum a large urn was pulled out, in which her beautiful hair could be seen with part of her head where there was still some attached. Since I saw several people pulling hand-fuls of hair from this urn, I followed their example and wrapped them like a relic in paper. I still have enough of it to make a wig, which I offer you with all my heart.

The peregrinations of Agnès Sorel's remains were not yet over. On June 9, 1795, the delegate Pochol had the urn exhumed, took the hair that re-mained and broke the jaw to extract the teeth, which several people di-vided among themselves, before putting everything back in the same spot. On December 16, 1801, de Pommereul, State Councillor and prefect of Indre-et-Loire, had the urn exhumed and deposited it at the subprefec-ture's offices, where it remained until 1809. During that time, the mau-soleum was restored and placed in the royal residence. The final exhu-mation occurred in 1970 in order to undertake a new restoration of the mausoleum and to place it somewhere more accessible to the public: the royal castle of Loches.

In 2005, the general council of Indre-et-Loire wished to reestablish her tomb in the collegiate church of Saint Ours, as much for museological reasons as to respect the last wishes of the deceased. On this occasion, we were asked by both Jean-Yves Couteau, of the General Council of Indre-et-Loire, and Pascal Dubrisay, elected official of the town of Loches, to conduct a scientific analysis of the remains of Agnès Sorel, to check their authenticity, and if possible, to define the causes of her death.

When the funerary monument was lifted, the urn of Puisaye sand-stone, dating to the 18th century, was indeed present. An initial X-ray examination at the university hospital of Lille confirmed the presence of human remains, arranged in several stratigraphic layers. The bones in the urn were generally very fragmented and crumbly, which made them difficult to identify. Fragments of face and mandible were recognizable, but only ten to fifteen percent of the whole skeleton was preserved. Also present were plant remains (leaves, seeds, twigs) that came from flowers initially present on the body of the deceased, and some remains of a prob-able internal embalming, as well as some rubble and metallic fragments. Remains of sarcophagus insects were also sampled and identified. Inside the urn, the bones were distributed in an orderly way, from the feet to the head, which was placed on top of all the rest. Some teeth were found, showing only minor wear, an absence of caries, and no striations indica-tive of dental enamel hypoplasia. Some hair was also brought to light.

It was difficult to determine the sex of the subject with certainty based on the examination of the bones, even though the majority of the criteria were female. The same is true for the age of the subject. In fact, there was much uncertainty regarding the date of birth of Agnès Sorel. The years 1409 and 1422 were the most commonly put forward. On this point, the minor wear of the teeth and absence of vertebral arthritis provided good arguments in favor of an estimated age between twenty and thirty years, which would preclude a date of birth for Agnès Sorel in 1409, as some his-torians had initially suggested. A more detailed analysis of the teeth gave an average age at death of between twenty-three years and nine months and twenty-seven years and nine months. The year of birth of Agnès Sorel thus wavers between 1422 and 1426.

Small amounts of dental tartar were present, demonstrating the excellent dental hygiene of the subject. Its microscopic examination showed a mixed diet consisting of meats and vegetables, which would correspond with that of a person of high rank. Joël Blondiaux counted the rings of dental cement, which evidenced the possibility of a minimum of three pregnancies; this tallies with the biographic notes on Agnès Sorel, who gave Charles VII three daughters (Charlotte, Marguerite, and Jeanne), and a fourth child who survived for only a short time. That last birth, just a few days before the death of Agnès Sorel, does not show on the subject's teeth, the mineralization of dental cement being slow and delayed.

The hair found was black, but this pigmentation was artificial and resulted from an attack by the lead sarcophagus that produced a *post mortem* deposit on the surface. Its natural color was blond. Examination of the hair under polarized light showed a twisting, characteristic of hair pulled back or to the side, and curled. According to Marine Cotte and Joël Poupon, our patient's hair contained high levels of mercury in the centre, along with lead on the surface, probably deposited during the body's time in the coffin. Unfortunately, no useable DNA could be extracted from the remains of this patient.

Analysis of the putrefaction fluid still present in the urn and on the bones allowed Françoise Bouchet to diagnose an infection of roundworm (small whitish worms) in the subject's intestines, a very common disease at that time. Recommended remedies consisted of an intake of mercury, sulfur, or salt taken with medicinal fern.

And so to the big question. What did Agnès Sorel die of, since everything suggests that we really are dealing with her? In her organic remains, we found traces of male fern that were used to treat worms. But in strong doses, its use can lead to fatal poisoning. The recovered spores of male ferns do not allow us to say whether she was poisoned by ingesting them in a therapeutic context.[1] On the other hand, mercury (or quicksilver as it was known at the time) found in large quantities in the center of the hair could be considered as a potential cause of death. Mercury had also been found in the body's putrefaction liquid, as well as within some skin fragments. There is no doubt that this heavy metal, which does not occur naturally in the human body, came from a medicinal prescription intended to cure her roundworms. It was not deposited *post mortem*, and was therefore present in the body of the deceased when she died.

Did Agnès Sorel die as a result of her treatment, or was she poisoned? The mercury in her hair is distributed longitudinally, which is logical in itself if this was a chronic treatment. Yet the presence of mercury *at the roots* of Agnès Sorel's hair is much too great to be considered a therapeutic dose (the concentration was 10,000—in fact, 100,000 times the therapeutic dose!) In all likelihood, Agnès Sorel died of an acute fatal poisoning, a brutal overdose by ingestion. But was this murder? Even if this hypothesis seems the most plausible, a therapeutic accident should not be excluded (an accidental overdose of mercury), nor a suicide. Agnès Sorel had just lost her fourth child, and at the time of her death her position at court was no longer so secure. Charles VII was interested in another young woman, and it is not impossible that Agnès Sorel would have preferred death to disgrace.

But if it was murder, who could have held a grudge against "la belle Agnès"? From this point of view, the most frequently mentioned trail is that of the Dauphin of France, the future Louis XI, who had a stormy relationship with his father's favorite, though it is hard to image the prince poisoning his enemy himself. Accomplices must have taken care of the sinister task. Who were they? For a long time, historians accused Jacques Coeur. But Agnès Sorel counted among his most faithful supporters. What would he have gained by eliminating her? In any case, during his trial, he strenuously denied any involvement in the poisoning, and was in fact acquitted on this point. Another possibility is Robert Poitevin, Agnès Sorel's personal physician, who had access both to the patient and to mercury. . . . But was he even present at Jumièges at the time of the events? Other trails are possible. In the history of France, Agnès Sorel has a special place because she is considered to be the first "official favorite" of a king of France. Far from being satisfied with seducing Charles VII, Agnès Sorel played a major political role during her years at court beside her lover through troubled times: the Hundred Years' War was not yet over. The interference of the "Dame de Beauté" in the kingdom's affairs must have earned her some resentment, which was perhaps the reason for her demise. Who killed Agnès Sorel? Unfortunately, we will probably never know.

\* \* \*

This analysis of Agnès Sorel's remains also allowed us to rebuild her face, based on the remains of the cranium found in the urn. Having digitized the contours of the bones and added the known details of the subject (sex, age, anthropometric indicators, etc.) a computer model was made by J.-N. Vignal, of the Institut de recherche criminelle de la gendarmerie nationale (forensic science department of the French National Gendarmerie), to see what the person considered to be the most beautiful woman in the kingdom looked like. Subsequently, we compared the scan of the cranium and the reconstruction of the face with the bust "said to be Agnès Sorel" when she was Isabelle of Lorraine's lady-in-waiting, today kept in the museum of Berry de Bourges. The superposition shows a perfect anatomical match between the cranium and the bust of Agnès Sorel. We did the same thing with her effigy, made just after her death by an unknown sculptor, which is preserved at Loches. Once again, the superposition of the cranium and reconstructed face is perfect, with the exception of the tip of the nose, mutilated by the blows of the revolutionaries and later remade.

\* \* \*

To finish, we inventoried a dozen strands of hair of the "Dame de Beauté" held in public and private collections. From this group, eight strands were examined under a binocular optical microscope, then compared with a sample from the funerary urn. The results are definitive: all the hair had the same diameter, the same shape, the same natural color (ash blonde) and the same blackish deposit on the surface. Seven of these samples contained particles of gold from the golden mantilla that held back Agnès Sorel's hair when she was buried. Thus, everything pleads in favor of the authenticity of these "relics" of Agnès Sorel.

As we can see, the study of this funerary urn has taught us a lot about the life and death of Charles VII's favorite. Whether she was assassinated or died accidentally, Agnès Sorel rests once again in the collegiate church of Saint Ours of Loches. A visitor passing through the town who stands in front of her magnificent effigy can admire her radiant beauty, forever frozen in white marble.[2]

## Notes

1. It should be noted that male fern has never been used for embalming which, in principle, excludes its presence for this purpose.

2. See P. Charlier, "Qui a tué la dame de Beauté ? Étude scientifique des restes d'Agnès Sorel (1422–1450)," *Histoire des sciences médicales*, 40/3, 2006, pp. 255–263; P. Charlier, J. Poupon, F. Bouchet, J. Blondiaux, M. Cotte, A. Cotten, J.-N. Vignal, V. Mazel, P. Georges, S. Bohic, C. Brombacher, E. de Dreuzy, P. Dubrisay, S. El-Balkhi, S. Harter-Lalheugue, I. Huynh-Charlier, C. Keyser, M. Le Bailly, B. Ludes, D. Morillon, P. Richardin, B. Sendid, J. Susini, X. Trufaut, Y. Van Der Plaetsen, F. Wallet, "Étude ostéo-archéologique des restes d'Agnès Sorel (Loches, Indre-et-Loire)," in P. Charlier (ed.), *Deuxième colloque international de pathographie, op. cit.*, pp. 419–526; P. Charlier, L. Brun, "Une parasitose endémique médiévale," *Annales de pathologie*, 30/2, 2010, pp. 160–162.

# IV

# RENAISSANCE TO MODERN TIMES

# 34

# QUEEN OF HEARTS

Diane de Poitiers (1499–1566)

In anticipation of her death, Diane de Poitiers wrote her will in 1564, and ordered a black-and-white (her favorite colors) marble tomb with her arms and devices in the church of Anet. Her heart was to be removed from the body, prepared and placed next to her husband, the Grand Sénéchal of Normandy, in the cathedral of Rouen. At her death, in 1566, her wishes were respected; the heart was prepared and sent to Rouen, while the body was embalmed, probably by the famous surgeon Ambroise Paré, who had looked after Diane de Poitiers when she had broken her leg falling from a horse the previous year. Unfortunately, the funerary chapel was still being built, so her funeral was held in the parish church of Anet, where her remains would stay for eleven years. It was only in 1577 that the mortuary chapel, built according to the plans of Claude de Foucques, was completed and that Diane de Poitiers could finally be buried with great pomp under the magnificent marble tomb attributed to Peirre Bontemps. Diane de Poitier's coffin was placed in a brick vault, and the tomb monument was placed above it. Five steps lead down into a vault six feet (1.8 m) high, twelve and a half feet (3.8 m) long and five and three-quarter feet (1.75 m) wide.

As for many other aristocrats, Diane de Poitiers' eternal rest would be short-lived. On June 18, 1795, some revolutionaries entered her mortuary vault, gutted the wooden envelope, took the lead coffin to make "patriotic bullets" from it, and defiled the cadaver, which had stayed in excellent condition, still with her formal dress. The naked body was then dumped on the lawn with the two small corpses buried beside her, her grand-daughters who had died young, also well-preserved, which the revolutionaries hastily identified as the children of Diane, resulting from her affair with her royal lover. But after a few days exposed to the air, the bodies began to decompose, and they were all thrown into a communal pit, dug beside the apse of the church. As is often the case on such occasions, the witnesses present took the opportunity to collect some pieces of clothing and some strands of hair of Henri II's bygone mistress. In 1884, a commemorative funerary monument was placed by the apse of the church of Anet, in the location traditionally held to be the ultimate burial place of Diane de Poitiers.

On May 24 and 25, 2008, with the permission of the mayor and municipal council of Anet, the communal pit at the foot of the monument erected in the late 19th century in the cemetery surrounding the parish church was reopened in an attempt to find the remains of the Grande Sénéchale. The search revealed eight skeletons, two of which were children. The bones were exhumed, individualized and sent to the hospital of Garches for analysis, with the aim of potentially identifying the remains of Diane de Poitiers. Only one skeleton might correspond to that identity, but only thirty to forty percent of that skeleton remained.

The first elements of authentication were brought to light by using forensic science techniques. In the absence of pelvic bones, only the mandible could establish that this was probably a female individual. The subject's vertebrae presented lesions caused by severe arthritis, and serious tooth loss allowed the age of the subject to be evaluated as being over forty-five years (Diane de Poitiers most probably wore dentures). The subject's left inner ear (petrous temporal) looked inflamed, lesions that are generally found as a result of chronic immersion of the head in cold water. Indeed, Diane de Poitiers swam extensively in the water courses around Anet, and did so until an advanced age. An ancient leg fracture (well-healed, incidentally) was found, which would correspond with the one sustained in 1565.

The toxicological analysis of Diane de Poitier's hair preserved in the castle of Anet (which came from the desecration of 1795) showed a gold content 250 times higher than normal. Such levels are particularly toxic, notably to the kidneys and bone marrow, and can cause death more or less rapidly. This high concentration was also evident within the intracranial deposits of solidified putrefaction fluid, thereby confirming at the same time the authenticity of the bones. The presence of this gold in the bones of Diane de Poitiers is not in itself surprising: for a long time her doctors had prescribed her gold salts so that she could preserve her eternal youth. . . . Some traces of quicksilver (mercury) were also detected in the hair and bodily putrefaction fluid, at toxic, but not lethal, doses.

Jean-Michel Duriez (the "nez" or nose for Jean Patou and Rochas) carried out an olfactory study and detected several scents: the fruitiness of formaldehyde, very light balsamic resin, vanillin, balm, and oak cask (damp wood). The first ingredient could be linked with the container of the sample smelled (a flask from a hospital), while the other scents are compatible with the containers and/or contents of the body after preparation. The toxicological analysis confirmed the presence of traces of lead on the surface of the bones, most probably resulting from a gradual contamination from the coffin over time.

But the most important, and paradoxically the most puzzling, information was the Carbon-14 date, which wavered between 900 and 1040 AD! This was the only detail that was theoretically discordant in this authentication of the remains of Diane de Poitiers. It was Professor Jean-François Saliège who found the key to the mystery: this anomaly of dating is a result of the aging of the samples due to the embalming products that were used, some of which are of fossil origin (bitumen, balm, aromatic oils, etc.). Although the Carbon-14 dating turned out not to contribute to the process of identification, at least it confirmed the existence of embalming with the addition of exogenous organic materials.

Taken together the elements discovered meant that the remains could be authenticated as being those of Diane de Poitiers and her two grandchildren. Henceforth, nothing prevented the inhumation, again with great pomp, of Diane de Poitiers in the chapel of the castle of Anet, within the original vault, where she now rests—we hope for her sake—for eternity.[1]

## Note

1. See P. Charlier, J. Poupon, I. Huynh-Charlier, J.-F. Saliège, D. Favier, C. Keyser, B. Ludes, "A Gold Elixir of Youth in the 16th Century French Court," *British Medical Journal*, 339, 2009, pp. 5311–5312 and P. Charlier, J. Poupon, I. Huynh-Charlier, J.-F. Saliège, D. Favier, J.-M. Duriez, A. Embs, C. Keyser, B. Ludes, "Diane de Poitiers (Anet): étude ostéo-archéologique," in P. Charlier (ed.), *Troisième colloque international de pathographie (Bourges, avril 2009)*, Paris, De Boccard, 2011, pp. 339–362.

# 35

# THE KING'S BODY

The Embalming of the Kings of France
(16th to 18th Centuries)

From birth to death, the daily life of the kings of France was governed by an etiquette that placed their existence under the permanent eye of the Court and its courtiers. The same was true for their inhumation. At the death of the sovereign, his body would be autopsied and then embalmed before being buried in Saint Denis, next to his predecessors. However, unlike the Etiquette, which codified all aspects of court life, no rule, no particular protocol governed the embalming process of the sovereign, which would evolve over the centuries according to events and practices.

The body of the king of France, chief of state, crowned prelate and descendant of Saint Louis, was traditionally preserved from "rotting" in anticipation of the resurrection promised by the Church. If this practice, which came from Egypt, answered a spiritual need, then its objective was also to delay the process of putrefaction as much as possible to mask any potential bad smells during the display of the body and its transfer and inhumation in Saint Denis. Charles IX, for example, had waited one and a half months to be interred. . . . But the conditions for embalming were not always straightforward. In some provinces, there was no embalmer of quality to be found. The unsuccessful embalming of Catherine de Medici, who died and was buried in Blois, a town with few appropriate drugs and spices, was the cause of some olfactory discomforts. . . .

Since Charles IX, when the king died, the body was autopsied by an elder of the Faculty of Medicine. Done in public under the scrutiny of the deceased's closest servants but to the exclusion of the royal family, this autopsy was a forensic act. Its aim was to confirm the identity of the deceased and to establish the cause of death, whether suspect or not. The operation consisted of a long incision from the sternum to the pubis in order to catalogue the organs present and to describe their condition. Then the body was given to the surgeons, who prepared the corpse for embalming. At the court of the French kings—unless clearly countermanded by the king when alive—they followed the tradition of the separation of the cadaver: one grave for the body, another for the heart and a third for the entrails (viscera). The body was emptied of all organs that could putrefy, the stomach, liver, spleen, brain, kidneys, and intestines, as well as the tongue and eyes, and these were put in a sealed barrel near the body, in a lead coffin. Only the heart was set apart, embalmed, and placed in a special reliquary.

The embalming of the kings of France is attested since the Carolingians, even if the embalming must have been only external, in order to maintain as presentable an appearance of the deceased as possible until his inhumation. The oldest known case is that of King Philippe I, who died in 1108 and was interred in Saint Benoît sur Loire (which allowed his remains to escape defilement in 1793). Exploration of his tomb showed that the body had been embalmed, but without a craniotomy. In those days, embalming was done by the court cooks, these latter being used to carving cold meats, stuffing them, and draining the blood. Only gradually did surgeons replace them, often accompanied by apothecaries or chemists to help them in their task. But doctors were never embalmers; they considered the practice to be unworthy of their profession and so left it to others.

King Louis IX died of dysentery on August 25, 1270 outside Tunis, during the Eighth Crusade. This raised the issue of embalming and transporting his body. A power struggle then began over the corpse—and the prestige of owning it—between Charles of Anjou, King of Sicily and brother of Louis IX, and his nephew Philip III, the new king of France. An agreement was finally reached between the relatives: the viscera of Louis IX were placed with his brother, in the Abbey of Monreale, near Palermo, where they are still. The heart had been removed and placed in a reliquary. We do not know where it is today; perhaps in the Sainte-Chapelle? Or did it subsequently disappear completely? To begin with, the embalmers had attempted to preserve the body. But the corpse, put in wine, went sour. . . .

Only the ultimate solution remained. The body was cut up and boiled until the flesh became detached and the bones could be retrieved. And so the bones of the dead king crossed the Mediterranean, and he was buried at Saint Denis on May 22, 1271. Relics of Louis IX must have stayed in Tunisia, such as pieces of skin or other parts of the body, but we do not know where they are today. Considered to be a saint during his lifetime, Louis IX was canonized in record time on August 4, 1297. The grave of the body of Saint Louis was then opened to extract some relics, which were exhibited in various parts of the country. The rest was defiled by the Protestants. By the time of the defilement of 1793, all that remained of the king was one phalanx!

As we have seen before, the body of Agnès Sorel was embalmed. So too were those of Louis XI (1483) and Charlotte de Savoie (1483), interred in the church of Notre Dame de Cléry Saint André (Loiret), whose heads also underwent a craniotomy. The study of these two patients has provided a better understanding of how French sovereigns were embalmed. To help him in his task, the embalmer used the *rigor mortis*, the rigidity of the corpse, like a third hand when sawing the cranium, either at the time of the autopsy or of the embalming. The aim was to extract the brain to study it (mainly to look for a cause of death), as well as to put aromatic substances in the cranial cavity, and to preserve the face as well as possible.

In the case of Henry IV, the objective of his autopsy was to determine which organs had been touched by Ravaillac's weapon, as is related by the king's surgeon, Jacques Guillemeau:

One wound is on the left side between the armpit and the breast, on the second and third rib from the top, the entry of which is the width of a finger, running on the pectoral muscle, toward the breast for the length of four fingers without penetrating beyond the chest. The other wound is lower down, between the fifth and sixth rib, in the middle of the same side, the entry of which is two fingers wide, penetrating the chest and piercing one of the lobes of the left lung and from there cutting the stem of the venous artery, in which one can put a little finger, slightly below the left auricle of the heart; from this place, both lungs pulled blood, which they threw in floods through the mouth, and were so filled with the excess that they became all blackened as if bruised. Also found was a large quantity of coagulated blood in the chest, and also some in the right ventricle of the heart, all of which caused the large vessels leaving it to be distended with blood: and the vena cava to the right of the blow (very close to the heart) appeared blackened from the contusion made by the point of the knife. All judged that this wound was the sole and necessary cause of death. All other parts of the body were found whole and healthy, like all bodies of very good temperance and of very fine structure.

The embalming of Henri IV (1610) would be done according to the "art of the Italians," probably on the orders of his wife, Marie de Medici. Henri IV's cranium would not be sawed, and as the reader will discover in the next chapter, this detail is of some importance. The official report of the embalming of his successor, Louis XIII, tells us about the products used. Once the body was autopsied and the viscera removed, the corpse was cleaned using balsamic vinegar containing cloves, roses, lemon, orange, colocynth, styrax, and balsamic resin. Cotton balls filled the eyes, mouth, nose, and ears. The body was then filled with several balms intended to prevent putrefaction and to mask bad smells. Among the products used were cypress bark, lavender, thyme, sage, rosemary, salt, pepper, absinth, balsamic resin, styrax, myrrh, oregano, cinnamon, dill, cloves, lemon peel, aniseed, and incense. Once filled, the body was sewn up and could be displayed. The vast range of ingredients used and their onerous rarity limited the practice of embalming to the high French aristocracy. This had not escaped Voltaire, who would write:

> Herodotus and Diodorus report that there were three sorts of embalming, and that the most expensive cost one Egyptian talent, evaluated over a hundred years ago at 2683 French pounds, and which, as a consequence, would today be worth more or less double. This honor was not given to poor people. With what would they have paid it, especially in those times of famine? The kings and grandees wanted to triumph over death itself; they wanted their bodies to last eternally [ ... ]. Thus the bodies of great lords had to be preserved preciously, so that their souls could find them again: but no-one cares for the souls of the people; they were simply made to work in the tomb of their masters.[1]

There were exceptions to being embalmed. For example, Anne of Austria (1688), wife of Louis XIII and mother of Louis XIV, asked expressly, a little before she died of breast cancer, that only her heart be removed, "without any other openings," so that it could be taken to the chapel of the Coeurs du Val de Grâce. As a result, the body was not autopsied, and if there was any embalming, it was only external, before the body went on to the basilica of Saint Denis. Sometimes, state reasons could overrule personal considerations. Such was the case of Henrietta of England (1670), who was autopsied at the behest of Louis XIV to stop rumors of poisoning. When the opening of the body was virtually over, the cranium and the "organs of generation" were left intact to respect the modesty (and beauty?) of the deceased.

Louis XIV would be the last French sovereign of the 18th century to be embalmed when he died in 1715. Like those of his predecessors, his remains were dispersed in various locations. The entrails and brain of the king (as well as those of Louis XIII) were sealed under the steps leading to the altar in the cathedral of Notre Dame de Paris. Continuing the tradition introduced by Louis XIII, Louis XIV in turn willed his heart to the Jesuits and had it placed at the church of Saint-Paul-Saint-Louis in the Marais (today, all of them are in Saint Denis).

His distant successor Louis XV would not have the same considerations. Due to the risk of infection by smallpox, doctors opposed his autopsy and embalming. The corpse of the king was wrapped in strips in
order to protect those charged with transporting and burying him. Placed
in a lead coffin, the body of the king was driven by night to Saint Denis.

> The death of the king had definitely lost its character as a magical event
> and his body had lost some of its sacredness in favor of the necessities
> of public health, even though Louis XV could have been autopsied and
> embalmed by doctors who had been inoculated. But the king's small-
> pox was well-timed: deconsecration or not, this time the sovereign
> died like a modern man and not like a very Christian king, like a simple
> individual and not like a pontiff [ ... ]. Times had changed, as had the
> symbolic relationship with death and power.[2]

Even the monarchy had become mortal. This state of things was the pre-
cursor to the political convulsions that would sweep it away a few years
later.

At his death (1824), Louis XVIII would be the last king of France to be
autopsied and embalmed. This is an exceptional case, since we have both
the written report of the autopsy and that of the embalmer. Pharmacist
Labarraque first sprayed the cadaver with a soda solution in order to get
rid of the horrible smell of putrefaction emanating from it (mainly due
to gangrene). The rest of the procedure was fairly similar to that of his
ancestors: removal of the heart and viscera, cleaning of the body and fill-
ing with various substances, with improved techniques (the presence of
chemical products unknown under Louis XIV) and the presence of more
pharmacists in the process. It would, theoretically, be possible to judge
the effectiveness of this preservation: the body has not been maltreated
by revolutions and wars, and is still present in the crypt of the basilica of
Saint Denis, ready to be examined by future scientists. . . .

With the exception of Louis XVIII, buried after the Revolution, the
French sovereigns did not enjoy eternal rest. On August 1, 1793, from the
tribune of the National Convention, Deputy Barras ordered the destruction of the mausoleums of Saint Denis with this argument: "Pride and
royal prosperity seem still, even in the grave, to boast of faded grandeur.

The mighty hand of the Republic must efface unpityingly these superb epitaphs and demolish these mausoleums that would recall the frightening memory of the kings." The first defilement happened in August 1793, but the greater defilement occurred during the first half of October: the royal tombs of the basilica of Saint Denis were opened and desecrated. If the revolutionaries were motivated by the desire to efface the memory of their ancient masters, a more practical reason also guided them: to retrieve the lead sarcophagi to make "patriotic bullets" for the armies of the young republic. In fact, a foundry was built within the basilica itself, and it would be in use for many weeks.

The Convention sent commissioners to Saint Denis to oversee the smooth running of the operation. Among them was a certain Alexandre Lenoir (1761–1839), who was to play a very important role during these macabre days. In Saint Denis, the coffins were methodically opened one by one. Some bodies were exhibited before being put in the communal pit. Henri IV's coffin was opened on October 12: witnesses reported that "the preserved body was easily recognizable. Until Monday 14th, it remained exhibited in its shroud, and everyone was at liberty to come and look at it." Louis XIII was also exhumed and those assisting noted that his mustache was well preserved. Louis XIV suffered the same destiny and was found to be black "as ink," the presumed consequence of his gangrene. As for Louis XV, the last to arrive in the basilica, "released from all that wrapped him, he immediately fell into putrefaction, and such a disgusting odor came from him that it was not possible to stay there."

During all the profanation, Alexandre Lenoir played an ambiguous role. During this revolutionary fury, he safeguarded the effigies of the kings and transferred them to the convent of the Petits Augustins (today the École Nationale des Beaux-Arts), which would become the Museum of French Monuments on September 1, 1795. The public was then able to wander among the effigies, organized in chronological order. But at the same time as he was participating in saving these works of art, Alexandre Lenoir was able to satisfy his passion for famous human remains, which he collected. He had been spotted near Parisian cemeteries and the church of Saint Germain des Prés, in the quest for remains of Boileau and Descartes. . . . His most infamous exploit was the exhumation of the remains of Abelard and Héloïse in their coffin at Nogent sur Marne. Always short of money, Alexandre Lenoir sometimes even sold pieces to other collectors. As strange as it may seem to us today, this cult of relics, even profane ones, was not unusual in the 18th century. The ransacking of the royal tombs in the basilica of Saint Denis (and other graves) allowed him to increase his collection considerably: a scapula of Hugues Capet, a femur of Charles V, a vertebra of Charles VII, a vertebra of Charles IX, a rib of Philippe le Bel, a rib of Louis XII, the lower jaw of Catherine de Medici, a tibia of Cardinal de Retz (and probably the mummified head of Henri IV), all identified by a piece of paper, but not necessarily all authentic! Alexandre Lenoir gave these bones to Mr. Ledru, his doctor friend, the mayor of Fontenay aux Roses, who used to show these "relics of kings" to his most illustrious visitors.

In 1834, at the death of Mr. Ledru, his widow inherited the relics and gifted them in turn to her nephew, one Lemaire, without admitting to their origin, but recommending that he keep them very carefully. At the death of Mrs. Ledru, the said Lemaire discovered the importance of the "gift," and after keeping them for several years, he decided to will them to the state. Napoleon III then ordered these bones to be interred once again in Saint Denis.

However, for unknown reasons, the remains were not buried and the "royal relics" were put haphazardly into a simple box, deep in the stores of the Louvre Museum. It was only in 1893 that an article in *Le Figaro* bitterly criticizing the government's lack of interest in these royal remains forced the administration to begin actively looking for them. In August 1893, on the decision of the Minister of Education, Art, and Religion, an oak crate was specially made for the last journey of these bones, which were once again buried in the basilica of Saint Denis. As the saying went under the Old Regime, "The king goes where he sees fit."[3]

## Notes

1. Voltaire, *La Bible enfin expliquée par plusieurs aumôniers*, in *Œuvres complètes de Voltaire*, Paris, Société littéraire et typographique, 1785, XXXIV, pp. 97–98, note, cited by S. Perez, *La Mort des rois*, Grenoble, Jérôme Millon, 2006.

2. S. Perez, *La Mort des rois, op. cit.*

3. See P. Charlier, "Les procédures d'embaumement aristocratique en France médiévale et moderne (Agnès Sorel, le duc de Berry, Louis XI, Charlotte de Savoie, Louis XIII, Louis XIV et Louis XVIII)," *Medicina nei Secoli*, 18/3, 2006, pp. 777–798; P. Charlier, R. Grilletto, R. Boano, D. Gourevitch, B. Galland, J.-P. Babelon, J. Perot, "Ouvrir un corps de roi: pourquoi, comment ? Le cas d'Henri IV," *La Revue du praticien*, 61/6, 2011, pp. 880–885; P. Charlier, P. Georges, "Techniques de préparation du corps et d'embaumement à la fin du Moyen Âge," in A. Alduc-Le Bagousse (ed.), *Inhumations de prestige ou prestige de l'inhumation ? Expressions du pouvoir dans l'au-delà*, Caen, CRAHAM, 2008, pp. 241–273; S. Gabet, "Alexandre Lenoir: sauveur ou profanateur de momies ?," in P. Charlier, L. Lo Gerfo (eds), *Le Miroir du temps. Les momies de Randazzo (Sicile, XVIIᵉ–XIXᵉ siècle)*, Paris, De Boccard, 2011.

# THE HENRI IV AFFAIR

The Mummified Head of "Good King Henry"

In 2010, a multidisciplinary team of about twenty scientists and historians co-authored an article in the *British Medical Journal* attesting to the authenticity of an embalmed head as being that of King Henri IV. Here is not the place to repeat the whole story of this discovery, which was the subject of numerous articles, books, and a TV documentary, but simply to recall that no fewer than twenty concordant scientific and historical arguments pleaded in favor of this authentication. Among the main ones, let us just cite that the subject has pale skin, that it is male, of mature adult age (Henri IV died aged fifty-seven); very poor dental condition, a skin lesion on the right nostril (like that represented on the king's portraits); a scar on the bone of the upper left maxilla (possibly linked to the attempted assassination by Jean Châtel in 1594); a pierced right earlobe (an earring is attested to in a portrait of the king—admittedly a late one—kept in Chantilly); a Carbon-14 date of between 1450 and 1650 (Henri IV died in 1610); etc. Subsequently, based on the mummified head and a medical scan of it, and in co-operation with Philippe Froesch, we proceeded with an objective facial reconstruction of the subject; it corresponded on every point with the iconography of "good king Henry." Henceforth, "the mass was said," to paraphrase the famous saying of the deceased—that is, the die had been cast. The weight of the arguments in favor of the identification was such that a mistake was no longer possible. This head was indeed the mummified head of Henri IV, purloined at the time of the ransacking of the tombs in Saint Denis. Historical inquiry confirmed the complete traceability from the theft by Alexandre Lenoir through to the present-day depository some two hundred years later. The publication of our article was greeted with interest by the international scientific community, to say the least, as well as by the general public. However, enthusiasm was not unanimous.

The main sources of contestation were Professor Joël Cornette (université Paris-X), the paleopathologist Gino Forniaciari (University of Pisa), and Philippe Delorme, journalist at *Point de vue/Images du monde*. In the absence of useable DNA at the time, the main obstacle, according to our gainsayers, concerned the sawing of the cranium. According to the embalming tradition for the kings of France, it was customary to saw the king's cranium to extract the brain and to fill the cavity inside with aromatic plants. In addition, Alexandre Lenoir, who was present at the exhumation in 1793, wrote that the cranium of King Henri had been sawed. Yet the mummified head was intact. These arguments were inadmissible for two reasons. Although, as we have seen in the previous chapter, Alexandre Lenoir was actually present when the tombs of Saint Denis were opened in October 1793, his text was published in 1801, long after the exhumation. What is more, his account is but a compilation of stories of other witnesses present that day, greatly embellished by his hand. Alexandre Lenoir cannot be reasonably considered as trustworthy. In particular, the sawing of Henri IV's cranium is not mentioned in any of the other contemporary accounts and inventories of the revolutionary defilement. . . . But, as we now know, Henri IV had been embalmed "according to the art of the Italians," who did not practice craniotomy, probably on instruction of his wife, Marie de Medici (who, on her death, would have her cranium sawed . . . ). In the course of our research, we have also found that craniotomy, frequent though it is, was absolutely not systematic at the court of the French kings. The case of Henri IV is not unique by any means.

There was a new development in the affair when we were able to do a genetic analysis on a sample of tracheal tissue, taken during a fiber endoscopy on the mummified head. Coming from a deeper area than other samples analyzed in Copenhagen (Niels Bohr Institute) and Strasburg (Forensic Institute), it was hoped that it would be less contaminated by lead: this was indeed the case. Not only was some DNA extracted, but it was also analyzed. It was then of interest to compare it with that of Henri IV's close descendants. And as it happens, a reliquary exists containing some blood said to be of "Louis XVI."

This reliquary is a gourd that has been in Italy for over a century and that, according to the inscriptions, contains a handkerchief soaked in the blood of Louis XVI at the Place de la Concorde (known as the Place de la Révolution at the time), on January 21, 1793. The piece has been studied by a team of Spanish geneticists in Barcelona, and the conclusions showed that it was male DNA, presenting genetic characteristics that could be compatible with those of Louis XVI. As part of the identification procedure of the mummified head, we decided to have these two DNAs compared. The analysis showed that there was a partial match between the two sequences. The differences noted could be explained by tiny variations that occurred over the successive generations between Henri IV and Louis XVI.

Our gainsayers then had additional research undertaken by comparing the results of the blood said to be from Louis XVI with samples of blood from the living descendants of the same family (one Bourbon and two Orleans). The laboratory results were definitive: the DNA was incompatible among the blood said to be from Louis XVI, the head of Henri IV, and the present-day descendants.

Our conclusions differ from those of our gainsayers: for us, it seems pointless to try to compare a genealogical tree with genetic traceability. Not only when more than ten generations separate the samples tested, but particularly when, in that line of descent, there are some complex characters like Philippe of Orleans (the famous "Philippe Égalité") whose kinship and paternity are extremely doubtful. . . . This result nevertheless gave us pause for thought. Together with Carlos Lalueza Fox, we carried out a virtually complete sequencing of the blood said to be of Louis XVI (which was much better-preserved than that of the embalmed head): it appeared that there was very little chance that the exterior morphology of the subject and his geographic origin could correspond with those of Louis XVI, whose aspect and origin are known fairly precisely. In fact, the phenotype found in the blood analysis shows that there is little chance that this individual had had blue eyes, blond hair, large stature, and a genetic and geographic origin in Eastern Europe and northern Italy, which was the case for Louis XVI. It seems most likely that this "relic" does not contain the blood of Louis XVI, making the partial compatibility between the blood said to be of Louis XVI and the head of Henri IV pure chance. Hence the interest in having conducted an interdisciplinary, and particularly an anthropological, study that, through the accumulation of those other criteria of identification and through historical inquiry, allow us to be sure of the identity of the mummified head.

At the present time, no serious scientific or historical argument has been formulated, either in France or abroad, that can refute the authenticity of the mummified head. Henceforth, the big question remains: What to do with this authenticated head of Henri IV? Should it be given a civilian burial? Redeposited in its original place of burial, the basilica of Saint Denis? Should it be put in a glass case in a museum and exhibited to the public? For reasons of respect for the human being (even dead—respect does not disappear after death), we do not think so. If a new inhumation were to take place, what religious rite should be used—that current in 1610, or the present-day rite? Is a mass needed, or a simple benediction? Should there be a national funeral, as would befit a chief of state who died 400 years ago? Who will make the decision? To whom does this mummified head belong? To the French state, the continuator of the monarchy, or to his descendants? And which descendants? The Bourbons? The Orleans? So many questions without answers.

As we can see, to decide on the matter is impossible for the moment, and only a collective of experts could allow a decision to be made on the future of these remains, or take a position regarding their scientific exploitation, while respecting the laws of bioethics and human beings in general. From a medical point of view—for it is indeed a question of medicine, even if it is forensic medicine—these remains, even though fragmentary, must be considered as a whole patient. They must be treated with the same humanity and the same care as any other subject. While waiting for the situation to resolve itself, the head of "good King Henry" has rested for nearly six years now in the safe of a Parisian bank. A rather sad sepulchre.[1]

## Note

1. See P. Charlier, S. Gabet, *Henri IV. L'histoire du roi sans tête*, Paris, Vuibert, 2013; P. Charlier, I. Olalde, N. Solé, O. Ramirez, J.-P. Babelon, B. Galland, F. Calafell, C. Lalueza-Fox, "Genetic Comparison of the Head of Henri IV and the Presumptive Blood from Louis XVI (Both Kings of France)," *Forensic Science International*, 226/1–3, 2013, pp. 38–40; P. Charlier, I. Huynh-Charlier, J. Poupon, C. Keyser, E. Lancelot, D. Favier, J.-N. Vignal, P. Sorel, P.-F. Chaillot, R. Boano, R. Grilletto, S. Delacourte, J.-M. Duriez, Y. Loublier, P. Campos, E. Willerslev, M.-T. Gilbert, L. Eisenberg, B. Ludes, G. Lorin de La Grandmaison, "Multidisciplinary Medical Identification of a French King's Head (Henri IV)," *British Medical Journal*, 341, 2010, p. 6805; P. Charlier, "La tête momifiée de Henri IV: une identification médico-légale," *La Revue du praticien*, 60, 2010, pp. 1474–1477; I. Olalde, F. Sanchez-Quinto, D. Datta, U. M. Marigorta, C.W.K. Chiang, J. A. Rodriguez, M. Fernandez-Callejo, I. Gonzalez, M. Montfort, L. Matas-Lalueza, D. Luiselli, P. Charlier, D. Pettener, O. Ramirez, A. Navarro, H. Himmelbauer, T. Marques-Bonet, C. Lalueza-Fox, "Genomic Analysis of the Blood Attributed to Louis XVI (1754–1793), King of France," *Scientific Reports*, 4, 2014, col. 4666; P. Charlier, C. Lalueza-Fox, C. Hervé, "La tête d'Henri IV. Identification et problématiques éthiques," *La Revue du praticien*, 63, 2013, pp. 289–293.

# 37

# AUTOPSY OF AN AUTOPSY

Official Report of an Autopsy in
Saint Nectaire (1765)

Old papers can hide unknown treasures. Such is the case of an unpublished manuscript from the 18th century, which was offered to me one day by a colleague: the official report of an autopsy carried out in Saint Nectaire. The document is a twelve-page manuscript *in quarto*, dated June 26, 1765, and carries the fiscal mark of the Auvergne (two sols). It concerns an autopsy done by Antoine Doumiol and Jean Capet, on the order of the bailiff of Saint Nectaire. The patient studied is Antoine Thomas, "servant on the estate of Lambre,"[1] who had received, on the preceding June 18, a "gunshot" in the left thigh; his age is not mentioned. He died at his place of work, and the aim of autopsy was to determine whether the cause of death was due to this wound, or whether there were other causes. As was often the case at the time, the autopsy was carried out at the home of the deceased.

The left thigh is examined first: "we did not find any rotting, or mortification, no pus." The autopsy continues with the viscera:

> The flesh being almost natural in color, we then proceeded to the lower abdomen, and we found all the viscera contained in this location in their natural state without any damage, deterioration or change of color, with the exception of the duodenum, which was slightly yellow.

Same for the lungs and heart, both found in good condition. The cranium is examined in turn: "We then sawed the cranium, examined scrupulously the membranes and the mass of the brain which we found to be a natural color, without congestion, inflammation or deterioration." Nothing in there either, yet one detail would attract the attention of the two doctors: "But we declare that we noticed a swelling and considerable inflammation of the throat, the tongue being very swollen, the palate and the tonsils were swollen and almost black." Doctor Capet then points out that, on June 24, he had been called to the bedside of the patient:

> At three hours after midnight, I found Antoine Thomas sweating abundantly with a violent fever, and swelling and inflammation of the throat. Having been unable to bleed him because of the sweating, I applied a topical medicine to him that did not calm the inflammation, and could not stop the progress of this illness, which was a veritable quinsy. The patient, who could barely speak, told me that the doctor must be sent for. The patient died before he arrived. From there, I, a doctor, inferred that since this illness had begun three days ago without Mr. Thomas having had himself treated, the progress of the inflammation became so considerable that the passage of air was entirely closed off, and the result was prompt suffocation, which is the real cause of death of Thomas.

This official statement, very detailed medically, relates the last days of the patient. Briefly, we can summarize it thus. June 18: Antoine Thomas is shot in the left thigh and receives some initial treatment. June 21: the illness appears. June 24, second consultation: abundant sweating, and death in the night. June 26: autopsy.

Reading this document, we can establish a modern diagnosis. Antoine Thomas died of acute pharyngolaryngitis, the asphyxia being explained today by the obstruction of the upper airways either by an inflammatory edema, or by the development of an infectious membrane.

However, study of the document reveals one particularity and two modern anomalies. The particularity is that this autopsy was done by two people, when there was no obligation to do so at that time. Today, it is strongly recommended that an autopsy be done with a minimum of two people (this is called the "duality of experts").

The first anomaly concerns the autopsy of the body, which was not carried out in the normal order. Generally, one begins with the cranium and continues with the chest and stomach. This order follows a forensic logic: to examine the brain, the body sometimes has to be turned over, which could lead to problems if the stomach is already opened. . . . In the case of this autopsy, the two doctors began with the thigh, probably because they assumed that it was there that the cause of death would be found. So be it.

The second anomaly is of an ethical nature. The document in question does not specify from where the "shot" came that wounded the patient, even if it had nothing to do—apparently—with the cause of death. Our two doctors do not seem to be specialized in autopsies, and their statement is not very meticulous. We do not know what the famous "shot" consists of. Was it a shot from a gun, or was Antoine Thomas wounded in the thigh by the recoil of his rifle? We do not know. It is clear that what our two practitioners wanted was to be sure of persuading the tribunal that they were absolutely not responsible for this death. This then raises a question of ethics: Is it normal that one of the two doctors (Capet) who treated the patient was also one of those undertaking his autopsy? Even if there is no reason to doubt the honesty of the two practitioners, and if this practice was common in the 18th century, it would have been more ethical if the body had been examined by other doctors, in order to avoid any possible conflicts of interest.[2]

## Notes

1. All citations are translated from the original document.

2. P. Charlier, D. Gourevitch, "Un procès-verbal inédit (Saint Nectaire, 1765). Étude technique et diagnostic rétrospectif," *Histoires des sciences médicales*, 43/3, September 2009, pp. 307–318.

# 38

# THE FACE OF THE INCORRUPTIBLE

Maximilien de Robespierre (1758–1794)

Together with Philippe Froesch, a specialist in facial reconstruction, we worked on the scientific reconstruction of the face of Robespierre. To achieve this, we worked on two moldings of the face of the "Incorruptible" that had been made *post mortem* by Marie Grosholtz, the future Marie Tussaud and founder of the eponymous wax museum in London. One copy of this death mask is kept at the Museum of Natural History of Paris, the other in the museum of Aix en Provence.

I participated in order to identify the possible diseases and to understand better the traumatic context of the death of Robespierre. Testimonies relating to the last months of Robespierre, by his friends in the Assembly and his doctor Joseph Souberbielle, provide some important information. At the end of his life, Robespierre was exhausted, slept very little, and devoted himself completely to his work. According to the testimonies that have reached us, his complexion was yellow, particularly around the eyes, he had nosebleeds at night, and ate a dozen oranges at each meal. Robespierre also had ulcers on his face and legs, and suffered from ophthalmic troubles. In other words, it was nearly a dying man who was guillotined on July 28, 1794, at the age of thirty-six.

All these symptoms suggest a retrospective diagnosis of sarcoidosis, an autoimmune disease that engenders eye problems and complications of the liver, which leads to a waxy complexion and skin nodules. It remained to be seen whether this disease was apparent on his face, as is often the case. On the death mask, on the left and right nostrils, we noticed some lesions that appeared in relief and corresponded exactly with cutaneous sarcoidosis. A scan of the death mask allowed us to know more about Robespierre. We were able to identify the negatives of well over a hundred lesions (fifty-nine on the right half of the face, eighty-five on the left side!), which corresponded to innumerable smallpox scars. We knew that Robespierre had suffered from it, but we had not realized its seriousness.

On the eve of his execution, Robespierre had been gravely wounded during his arrest at the City Hall of Paris, where he had taken refuge with his partisans. Until now, we did not know whether that was due to an attempted suicide to escape his enemies, or to a shot fired by the policeman Merda, during the scuffle that led to him being apprehended.[1] Shortly after the taking of the City Hall, two practitioners were summoned to examine the wound of the "citizen-traitor Robespierre." This examination of the patient is not the most detailed, but at least it informs us of the circumstances of his arrest. The official statement was published in the 19th century and has never been contested or called into question.

On the death mask, the scar of the pistol shot is not visible. The statement of the two experts tells us that the explosion occurred inside the mouth, and that it was serious, knocking out two teeth and fracturing the mandible, but on the outside, the wound was barely visible because the small exit hole was blocked by coagulated blood. Externally, only an edema on the left side was apparent, visible on the death mask, causing the face to be slightly asymmetrical. In any case, this study has authenticated the death mask, since it corresponds perfectly with the pathological descriptions reported for Robespierre.

The bigger question remains: suicide or accident? With the information at our disposal, the theory of an attempted suicide seems the more probable, but there is no absolute certainty. The forensic doctors who examined Robespierre had already noticed that Merda's weapon was not properly loaded. If the shot had been fired at a distance, the damage would have been different from that described by the two practitioners. The most plausible theory might be that Robespierre seized Merda's weapon and placed the pistol in his mouth. But the fact is that the weapon was not sufficiently loaded and the hurriedness of his action could have caused an explosion leading to considerable damage in his mouth, but not to his death.

The publication of this reconstruction of the face of Robespierre set off a fairly surprising argument, which says much about the place of this person in our historical heritage. The main controversy revolves around the dichotomy between our work and the revolutionary iconography that has come down to us. The face of Robespierre that we presented differs a lot from the paintings and sculptures of the Incorruptible. But did those works show the truth? Were they sincere? If we compare all the portraits of Robespierre, we observe large differences in the features of his face. When Robespierre's portraits were done, he already carried the marks of smallpox . . . which do not appear on any of the paintings, engravings, or sculptures. Everything suggests that they had been "idealized," perhaps with the idea of propaganda. After all, it would not be the first time that a painter had exaggerated the portrait of his model. . . .

The other attack concerned the authenticity of the death mask. For some, it seemed incongruous to make a death mask of Robespierre just after his execution. But let us not forget that when Robespierre had been examined by the two forensic doctors, they kept the teeth that had fallen from his mouth as a result of the shot and offered them as souvenirs to some of the people present. All in front of the patient! At that time, it was not unusual to "trade" in the relics of important men. We also have the testimony of Madame Tussaud, who made death masks of Louis XVI and Marie-Antoinette. So why not that of Robespierre? In addition, we have proof of the antiquity of the death mask of Robespierre, because it was drawn by Vivant Denon on the back of a sheet of paper dated to the late 18th century. This mask is therefore not a fake, and even less a 19th century creation, as some have suggested.

The third point on which we were attacked is regarding the gunshot wound, which is not visible in the reconstruction. In the present case, we are dealing with a death mask of the face—and not with a complete impression of the head—that ends just in front of the ears. As the

practitioners who examined Robespierre told us, the exit hole of the pro-
jectile was tiny, and a blood clot blocked any bleeding. As we mentioned
above, only the edema is apparent. The blood must have drained through
the mouth. Moreover, at the moment when Robespierre was executed,
the executioner removed the bandage that held his jaw, leading to significant bleeding from the mouth and a horrible scream from the victim.

But the most surprising and least scientific of the controversies came
from a man of politics, who saw in our reconstruction:

> A very unengaging head, if I can judge from the published photograph.
> An old ruse of iconography, for which I pay the price more often than
> is my turn: ugliness of face is supposed to reveal the ugliness of the soul
> [ . . . ]. On seeing the presumed mask of Robespierre, like many others,
> I quickly understood that it was one more episode in the ideological
> struggle on the meaning of the content of the Great Revolution. The
> makers of this farce did not skimp on the means of tricking everyone.[2]

It is an understatement to say that we were surprised by this all-out attack
on our work. In all scientific research processes, discussion is perfectly
normal, desirable, and enriching. But where this reaction is concerned,
we are going well beyond this framework.

Firstly, our intention was to make the most realistic portrait possible,
based on the medical texts in our possession and the death mask that has
come down to us, without any bias. In the absolute, medicine is only at
the service of the patients. The most worrying thing in this reaction is the
obscurantist belief, evoked by this politician, that the most beautiful ideas
should come only from beautiful people, and that the physically unpre-
possessing should be the seat of harmful ideas. It is surprising that such a
concept of the world—which perhaps goes back to the *kalos kagathos* of
the Greeks—should be taken up here by a prominent politician, elected
by the people. Even if this head of Robespierre does not correspond to an
ideal of beauty, does it make his writings less pertinent or prevent his formidable rhetoric from being admired? Are the theories of Stephen Hawk-
ing without scientific value because his physique does not conform to the
canons of ancient sculpture? Clearly not.[3]

## Notes

1. At the same moment, Le Bas committed suicide, while his older brother, Augustin Robespierre, was thrown out of a window.

2. "Du masque de Robespierre à celui de Jean-Marc Ayrault," www.jean-luc-melenchon.fr.

3. See P. Charlier, P. Froesch, "Robespierre: The Oldest Case of Sarcoidosis?," *Lancet*, 382/9910, 2013, p. 2068 and P. Charlier, P. Froesch, G. Cheylan, "Robespierre: the Oldest Case of Sarcoidosis? Authors' Reply," *Lancet*, 383/9923, 2014, pp. 1127–1128.

# 39

## RIGOR MORTIS

The Mummies of Santa Maria de Randazzo
(17th–19th Centuries)

In 2008, the church of Santa Maria de Randazzo, Sicily, was due to undergo refurbishment works. Imagine the surprise of the workmen when, during the course of their work in the crypt, the collapse of a wall revealed a closed room containing more than a hundred human crania, more or less well-mummified, as well as the bodies of children.

Preliminary scientific studies began not long after the discovery. The crypt contained ninety-two crania of male individuals, nineteen female ones, and twenty-four indeterminate (twelve immature and twelve incomplete). No mummification chamber was found in the crypt, and the presence of these crania is not mentioned in any writings. We do not know where these mummies were before they were collected together; the only certainty is that the bodies had indeed been mummified. Deposits of "putrefaction fluid" were found in various places on the crania, proof that some bodies had been deliberately sat up, or laid out either on their backs or on their stomachs, with the intention of facilitating the drainage of the remains. Straw was found in some crania, and through the study of the mummified children's clothes, the mummies could be dated to between the 17th and the very early 19th centuries. It only remained to determine why they were there. That was the mission given to Luiza Lo

Gerfo, a student of archaeology, who arranged the cooperation with my team.

This practice of mummification was not rare in Sicily. A dozen churches have the same characteristics and the mummies of Palermo are the most emblematic of them. Mummification was facilitated by the local microclimate. In fact, Sicily enjoys marine air (the wind is heavily laden with sea spray) associated with emanations of sulfur (much present in Randazzo at the foot of Mount Etna). The Randazzo mummies are mummies of the "intermediate" type, in other words the process occurs naturally, through "draining" of the corpse, with minimal human intervention. At the death of the individual, the family (generally from the elite) entrusted the remains to the Capuchin monks who were charged with this transformation and paid for their services. Among the possibilities offered them, the monks could suspend the body in the trees to desiccate. Another technique was to seat the deceased on a "pierced chair," or lay them out on a hollow bed and wait for all the fluids to descend naturally over time. After six months or a year, they collected the completely desiccated mummy. The mummies were then aligned in the crypt of the church and could be visited by the family—and even by tourists, in the early 19th century.

There was a double objective behind this transformation. On the one hand, it was a mark of humility: at his death, the deceased became a "vanity," a *memento mori* exposed in the nave of the church or in the crypt. It was a case of educating the faithful, to remind them that human life was not worth much:[1] "As you are now, so once was I, as I am now, so you must be." On the other hand, this transformation of the body in a holy place had a theological motivation: to facilitate the passage of the soul to paradise— a little like the medieval charnel houses.[2] In parallel, the monks prayed for the salvation of the deceased's soul.

These bodies were mummified until the mid-19th century. Some mummies had even been reworked at some point after their "manufacture;" their skulls were sawed and filled with rosemary. For unknown reasons, the bodies then began to deteriorate and were put into a communal pit. Only the crania were kept back, but as these also began to degrade, they were placed in a closed room where they were forgotten—until their accidental discovery in 2008.

The medical importance of this discovery was obvious. The significant number of patients allowed the various pathologies present to be studied. Thus, we discovered that many of the diseases had a professional origin: complete edentation of a pastry cook (air saturated in sugar depositing itself on the surface of the teeth, or constant tasting of dishes leading to repeated caries then multiple loss of teeth before the usual age), syphilis, metastasized cancer, healed trepanations on one cranium. . . . Patient after patient, it was thus possible to reconstruct the daily life of this little Sicilian village.[3]

## Notes

1. The erudite reader will have noticed that in a passage in *Journey to the End of the Night* by Louis-Ferdinand Céline, Robinson leads a visit to a crypt containing mummified bodies. This practice seems to have been common at a certain period.

2. See Chapter 27, above.

3. See P. Charlier, L. Lo Gerfo (eds), *Le Miroir du temps. Les momies de Randazzo (Sicile, XVIIe–XIXe siècle)*, Paris, De Boccard, 2011.

# 40

# DISTANT MUMPS

An Epidemic of Mumps in Polynesia
in the 19th Century

It all began with a figurine made of whale ivory from the 18th century, about five inches (12 cm) high, that had been brought back from Polynesia and is today kept in the Cambridge Museum of Archaeology and Anthropology. The object comes from the collection of Sir Arthur Gordon, who was the governor of the islands of Fiji around 1870. Originally it had been made on the isles of Tonga and given by the community chief of Sabeto (Fiji) to a Fijian doctor (*Maafu*) as remuneration for having healed him of a swelling in the neck. The practitioner took the figurine with him to his home in Nandi (on the island of Viti Levu) and dedicated it to Lalavatu, a local goddess, wife of the principle god of Nandi. He also built a temple for her and inaugurated a lineage of priests charged with perpetuating her cult. Local witnesses reported that a nasal voice sometimes emanated from the figurine, and that the goddess was particularly dangerous, having the power to make swellings grow on the sides of men's necks: some died from these growths; others, more frequently, died at war. Lila (an idiom close to the name of the divinity) was the name given by the Fijians to this epidemic brought by the Europeans in the 19th century.

This very succinct description of the symptoms (swellings on the lateral parts of the neck) suggests, not with absolute certainty but with a strong probability, a diagnosis of mumps, the consequences of which could be serious in this isolated population. It could lead to testicular complications (orchitis), seriously affecting the fecundity of native populations who were completely naïve regarding the virus, or to potentially fatal central neurological complications (meningitis and/or encephalitis), as described in the legend surrounding this divinity.

This is a new example of disruption of the environmental balance, not simply from sporadic contact with Europeans (in the 17th century, the duration of these contacts was too short and rare to allow the passage of an infectious pool from one human group to another), but from the later colonization in the 19th century (longer-term and on a much larger scale). Mumps, along with other western epidemics (measles, rubella, smallpox, etc.), not only caused considerable loss of human life, such as is described in the early 20th century by Victor Segalen in the *Immémoriaux* regarding the archipelago of Tahiti, but also caused a crisis in the birth rate, making the depopulation of the native tribes all the more serious:

People were getting thinner, like old people, then, their eyes shining, their skin viscous, their breath punctuated with painful hiccups, they died gasping for breath. Others saw their limbs stiffen, their skin dry out like the beaten bark of the tree we wear on feast days and, just like this bark, become desensitized and rough; black and colorless patches tattooed them with horrible marks; the fingers, then the toes, bent like the claws of a bird, would become dislocated, and fall off. They were sown as they walked. Bones broke in the stumps into little pieces. In spite of their missing hands, chipped feet, open eye sockets, their faces devoid of lips and nose, these poor people still moved among the living for many seasons, their carcasses already putrefied, yet not quite willing to die. Sometimes, all the inhabitants of a river bank, shaken with fevers, bodies burgeoning with reddish pustules, eyes dripping blood, disappeared as if they had battled with the spirits-who-go-in-the-night. The women were sterile, or their awful pregnancies aborted without benefit. Inconceivable harm followed furtive embraces, or the most indifferent of ruts.[1]

The concern of this story is to establish a link between a medical description, an artifact, and oral traditions that have come down to us. The statuette thus bears witness to a disease that was striking endemically at that time and that we had known about only through the testimony of travelers. Mumps is invisible on the skeleton, and only in-depth (paleo-genetic) studies can show its presence.[2]

## Notes

1. Victor Segalen, *Les Immémoriaux*, 1907.
2. See P. Charlier, L. Brun, V. Hoang-Opperman, I. Huynh-Charlier, "Une épidémie d'oreillons en Polynésie au XIX<sup>e</sup> siècle: un exemple de paléo-épidémiologie," *Feuillets de biologie*, 53(305), 2012.

# 41

## HEAD HELD HIGH

Shrunken Heads of the Jivaros and Tattooed
Heads of the Maoris

Never a month goes by without the question of the restitution of human remains to "first peoples" being brought up in the press and media. Today, the main demands concern the shrunken heads of the Jivaros (and Shuars) and the tattooed heads of the Maoris that are in national collections.

Since the procedures concern human remains, forensic scientists are automatically consulted for authentication. As a multidisciplinary team, we have developed a procedure for the authentication of Jivaroan heads (*tsantsa*), by working on about twenty artifacts from private and public collections, in Paris and in the provinces. The aim is to be sure, after analysis, that the restituted head is indeed authentic.

To achieve this, we established about fifteen criteria linked to the making of these shrunken heads. Each operation in the shrinking of a head by the Jivaros leaves specific traces that allow us to be sure of its authenticity. For example, not a fragment of bone remains (only desiccated skin should be left); the eyes and mouth are sewn up; hairs in the nose and ears are visible; there is a hole in the forehead for a cord to be passed through so that the head can be worn as a pendant; decorations may be added, such as some cloth or feathers; the skin is black or dark because the head has been smoked or exposed to coals; small crystalline formations are often present inside it, coming from the hot sand that had covered the head, etc.

These indicators allow real heads to be distinguished from fake ones. Over the years, fake Jivaroan heads have been made for "tourists" and travelers looking for exotic souvenirs. Some of these fake heads were made from animals—when it was not a case of the head of a Westerner slain by the tribe. . . . Some of these fakes have shown up in public collections. With this scientific process, it is now possible to disentangle the real from the fake and thereby to return authentic heads.[1]

The same problem occurs with the restitution of Maori heads. A forensic examination was undertaken on virtually all the heads in public collections in France prior to their official restitution to New Zealand. This work resulted in a better understanding of the process of Maori tattooing in order to gain the maximum amount of reliable information so as to be able to return them to the legitimate descendants. Maori facial tattoos provide a mini biography of the individual. The stages of life of the subject, as well as his personal qualifications, were represented by very detailed tattoos. For example, based on his facial tattoos, it was possible to deduce that a person came from the north of the archipelago, that he had lost his father, that he was a former chief, etc., thereby allowing the person he was speaking with to know with whom he was dealing, and to recognize the correct person at first sight.

But beginning in the 19th century, when such heads were stolen and sold to Westerners, some tattoos were added post mortem to increase their market value. For the Maoris, only ante mortem tattoos are valid. When a request for restitution is made, it is necessary to differentiate between the tattoos and to see whether they correspond with the area of origin of those making the request. During the authentication process, the forensic scientist must have access to the head to examine it with a binocular microscope, and all the tattoos must be examined one by one. Those made post mortem are recognized by their sharp edges, the absence of patina and the complete absence of scarring. At the end of our study, it transpired that one of the heads in the collections was covered only with post mortem tattoos. It will thus be very difficult (other than by using the molecular biology tool of DNA) to return it to its original clan.[2]

# Notes

1. P. Charlier, I. Huynh-Charlier, L. Brun, C. Hervé, GL de la Grandmaison, "Shrunken Head (Tsantsa): A Complete Forensic Analysis Procedure," *Forensic Sci Int*, 222 (1–3), 2012, pp. 1–5.

2. P. Charlier, I. Huynh-Charlier, L. Brun, J. Champagnat, L. Laquay, C. Hervé, "Maori Heads (Mokomokaï): The Usefulness of a Complete Forensic Analysis," *Forensic Science Med Pathol*, 10(3), 2014 pp. 371–379.

# EPILOGUE

These cases sweep across a very broad historical spectrum, from prehistory to the 19th century. Yet, far from being disparate and dispersed, they all follow the same methodology: that of casting a medical eye on bone remains to reconstruct, in an objective way, their state of health, their past activities and their cause of death. Placed side by side, these individuals build up a story: that of the evolution of mankind in his environment, and also of humans among humans.

What does the future hold for the discipline of osteoarchaeology? Perhaps especially interdisciplinarity—in other words, intense and fruitful collaboration with other fields and other scientific and humanist disciplines: forensic scientists, historians, archaeologists, anthropologists, and ethnographers. Exchanges are working so well that it would be legitimate, in the near future, to see an archaeologist testifying at the bar during a trial in criminal court, in the same way that a forensic scientist presents his or her latest work at a conference on Egyptology or Greek epigraphy. . . . Exchanges between university disciplines are not dispersion but emulation, progress. They are the only key to objectivity and scientific excellence, to the "demonstration of truth," as one says in court.

Richard the Lionheart, Agnès Sorel, Diane de Poitiers, Henri IV, Robespierre: so many patients, the study of whom has been useful for forensic anthropology because it led to the improvement of diagnostic techniques. Patients, the publication of whose cases will be able (we hope) to influence research in various subjects such as toxicology, facial reconstruction, radiology and so on.

However, we must not forget that these remains are those of real people, and not just archaeological objects or simple cases of experimentation. In the future, will we perhaps dig as many tombs or study as many mummies, but with the obligation of reburying them or of displaying them in a more sober, less spectacular way? The use of digital duplicates of human remains might perhaps be useful to continue work on cases once the remains have been interred again and have returned to dust. In all cases, we owe them respect—the same respect that we would wish for our own remains, when they are being studied a few centuries from now by our future colleagues. . . .

# APPENDIXES

# IS THERE A RISK OF INFECTION
# FOR PHYSICAL ANTHROPOLOGISTS?

What light can the forensic anthropologist shed on the risks of infection associated with the study of human remains?[1]

Very recently, a publication by Jean-Michel Claverie, Director of Research at the CNRS in Marseille, revived the debate on this "Pandora's box" of ancient biological remains (a direct reference to the new genus described by this researcher—the Pandoravirus—and its halo of unknowns . . . ). In March 2014, in the prestigious journal the *Proceedings of the National Academy of Sciences*, he describes having isolated some DNA viruses (which he calls *Pithovirus sibericum*) from deep in an ancient environment: frozen soil from Siberia nearly 30,000 years old.[2] The increasingly frequent genetic exploration of what are known as paleosols will lead to the discovery of unknown species of bacteria, viruses, and parasites whose potentially dangerous character could take hold . . . in theory.[3]

Why "in theory"? Because, in the great majority of cases, these infectious elements have absolutely no impact of human physiology. In addition, genetic studies require the soil to be sampled in a "sterile" way, in other words, without direct contact between the environment and the sample, which is analyzed only in a laboratory. The real danger—potential once again—comes from global warming and the melting of these paleosols, which have been frozen since the last ice age. This melting risks reactivating dormant infectious agents that have been forgotten by the human immune system for tens of thousands of years and that could be spread with the outflow of water.[4] Herein lies the value of understanding them well in advance, and of evaluating their potential dangerousness.

But is it dangerous to work on dead bodies? Are they still contagious postmortem? In theory, yes. Numerous viruses and bacteria are still detectable postmortem, but their contagiousness has perhaps not been evaluated very well, simply because it is not possible to undertake experiments in this domain. Thus we are reduced to following up case reports, which inform us more or less well on this professional and environmental risk.[5]

When performing any autopsy, for example, it is normal to wear as much protective clothing as possible: a gown, overshoes, plastic cap, several layers of gloves including cut-resistant gloves, mask, glasses, etc. Like in an operating theater, this is done so as not to contaminate the dead body with our own organic elements (hair, etc.), and also so as to not be contaminated by any infectious agents from the corpse. The dead body is, in fact, in the process of decomposition, even of putrefaction, and undergoes a massive multiplication of bacteria (postmortem flora and fauna). Death can also have been the consequence of an infection (by bacteria, virus, parasite, or prion), and it is important not to contaminate oneself when the "door is wide open" on pathological organs: the abdomen laid bare, lungs exposed to the air and cut on a glass plate only 40 cm from our own mouths, sawn cranium, with splashing of microparticles of blood and cerebrospinal fluid. . . . It is easy to imagine the professional risk run in the case of the autopsy of a patient with tuberculosis, or with H1N1 flu, or who died of meningitis.

For more ancient bodies, the risk is still not negligible. During a congress on funerary anthropology, an Italian colleague reported having excavated a crypt in a church containing some 16th-century mummies. While "unwrapping" one of them, he identified with his naked eye some skin lesions compatible with smallpox. He had to remain confined in the crypt with his team for hours—I think it was even for several days—long enough to determine whether the virus was still contagious or if time (and embalming) had rendered it inactive.

The danger can seem distant, but it is actually quite real. Anthropologists recount an "urban legend"—a completely false story, which testifies to the fascination that ancient germs hold and to their potential dangers. The story has it that in the 1990s, some scientists went to exhume the remains of explorers who had died in the Arctic of Spanish flu. Their bodies were found almost intact in the permafrost, but the virus was also intact, and the scientists died shortly thereafter . . . of Spanish flu.[6] This "legend" is, in fact, based on a 1998 expedition, by the Canadian Kirsty Duncan, to Spitzbergen, to exhume the bodies of seven miners who died in 1918 of Spanish flu and were buried in the permafrost. More seriously, other colleagues have approached dead bodies that were carriers of small-pox with absolutely no impact on their health, such as a team from Toulouse and Strasburg working on the corpse of a Siberian shaman, dead some 300 years.[7]

Do archaeologists take precautions when working on dead bodies? Generally, they exhume them with bare hands when they are excavating cemeteries, even if it is a cemetery for plague victims or lepers, because experience has shown that there is no risk of infection from these diseases. But any opening up of a confined space could be dangerous because an infectious agent could have proliferated and be suddenly released: this was how one of us caught an atypical mycobacterial infection while working on the funerary urn of Agnès Sorel. . . . And what can one say about Tutankhamun's tomb in which, according to some researchers, the quite unusual atmosphere and the presence of certain foods, balms, and textiles had favored the proliferation of *Aspergillus niger* or *flavus* (fungi incriminated, by the same researchers, in the famous curse of the Pharaohs, although *Pseudomonas* and *Staphylococcus* were also suggested as potential infectious agents).

Recently, at the request of the Musée de l'Homme, we worked on the potential danger of infection of the Olivier collection (put together in 1945), housed in the museum's old buildings on the Place du Trocadéro, in Paris. Forty-two skeletons, considered to be particularly slimy and oozing, were the subject of a bacteriological and mycological study through cultures on normal growth medium (CHU Paris-Ouest / Université de Versailles-Saint-Quentin-en-Yvelines): twenty-eight were sterile, while four were carriers of alpha-hemolytic streptococcus, four of coagulase-negative staphylococci, and six of non-specific bacilli. In short, banal floras within the dusty remains, no more dangerous than that found on any dirty surface.[8]

The paleopathology of smallpox was at the origin of an awakening of professional conscience regarding the potential dangers of dead bodies, particularly following the discovery of the mummy of the Pharaoh Ramses V, which was covered with a characteristic rash that has since been considered to be a typical case of smallpox in the ancient world. In his descriptive article, Dr. Zuckerman underlined that the risk of infection from ancient smallpox was minimal. Nevertheless, he recommended that all the archaeologists and anthropologists who had been in contact should be vaccinated—although, given what we now know, this vaccination should not be recommended systematically for such professionals because it, in itself, carries some real risks.[9]

Clearly then, the risk to anthropologists of professional exposure to infectious agents is largely theoretical. The only really contaminating germs are essentially of taphonomic origin and linked to the bacterial and mycological proliferation of decomposition/putrefaction. The universal rules in matters of hygiene seem to be sufficient, except in conditions of immunodepression or immunosuppression (subject to a personal evaluation by the occupational health service).

## Notes

1. Article published in *Feuillets de Biologie*, 319/55, 2014, pp. 63–65.

2. M. Legendre, J. Bartoli, L. Shmakova *et al.*, "Thirty-Thousand-Year-Old Distant Relative of Giant Icosahedral DNA Viruses with a Pandoravirus Morphology," *Proceedings of the National Academy of Science*, 3 March 2014.

3. P. K. Lewin, "Mummified, Frozen Smallpox: is it a threat?," *Journal of the American Medical Association*, 253/21, 1985, p. 3095.

4. J.-M. Claverie, C. Abergel, "Pithovirus: un virus géant venu du fond des âges," *Biofutur* 352, 2014, pp. 50–51.

5. P. Charlier, C. Hervé, "No Embalming for French HIV+: Ultimate Discrimination or Educational Issue?," *Anthropology* 1/2, 2013 (http://dx/doi/org/10.4172/2332-0915.1000103).

6. A. H. Reid, T. G. Fanning, J. V. Hultin, J. K. Tautenberger, "Origin and Evolution of the 1918 "Spanish" Influenza Virus Hemagluttinin Gene," *Proceedings of the National Academy of Science* 96/4, 1999, pp. 1651–1656; J. L. Davis, J. A. Heginbottom, A. P. Annan *et al.*, "Ground Penetrating Radar Surveys to Locate

1918 Spanish Flu Victims in Permafrost," *Journal of Forensic Sciences*, 45/1, 2000, pp. 68–76.

7. P. Biagini, C. Thèves, P. Balaresque *et al.*, "Variola Virus in a 300-Year-Old Siberian Mummy," *The New England Journal of Medicine*, 367/21, 2012, pp. 2057–2059.

8. P. Charlier, N. Gabrielli, "Les limites du nettoyage et de la restauration des restes humains anciens," *Conservation-restauration des biens culturels*, 25, 2007, pp. 25–28.

9. A. J. Zuckerman, "Paleontology of Smallpox," *The Lancet*, 1984/2, p. 1454.

# CAN SCIENCE BE IMMODEST?

"What is dead would not know how to die."
(A diviner from Abomey, Benin)

Should everything be published about research done on humans?[1] Should the application of fundamental principles such as consent, medical confidentiality, respect for the human body, and the right to one's image be stretched across time and space? Man is free, but responsible; which means that we cannot, must not say or show everything. Can science, which is supposed to be "impartial," handicap itself with modesty? Respect for the dignity of the individual does, in fact, include respect for his or her modesty.

We have read, over the past months and years, some unusual publications in peer-reviewed international biomedical journals, dealing with ancient skeletons and mummies. As an example, we saw the genealogical tree of Tutankhamun's family in the *Journal of the American Medical Association*[2] (with its load of incestuous relations revealed by genetic studies), a genital tumor—with supporting photo—on the mummy of Maria of Aragon, who died in 1568, in *The Lancet*[3], and numerous photographs of the mummy of Ötzi, that Neolithic man found in the Austro-Hungarian Alps, naked, with what remains of his genitals clearly visible.[4] Is this nudity justified by a method of conservation? Most probably not. . . . Are these publications motivated by a scientific approach, or by the curiosity of the researcher? Should such documents be divulged, in contradiction to the Hippocratic oath, according to which, "whatsoever I [the doctor] shall see or hear in the course of my profession, as well as outside my profession in my intercourse with men, if it be what should not be published abroad, I will never divulge, holding such things to be holy secrets."[5] So, one must ask the question: Should all or part of the intimate anatomy of people who disappeared centuries ago and who have been accurately identified be the subject of publications available across the world without any restriction?

False modesty? Superfluous questioning? Not at all. They were once people, even if only their skeleton or deteriorated mummy remains. But time does not efface everything: the code of ethics states that respect for the patient does not end with his or her death. As for the modified Law of Bioethics of 1994 (law no. 2011–814 of July 7, 2011), it protects persons subjected to experiments and scientific investigations, without establishing any time limit.

What about these publications? Are they scientific publications that fall within the framework of research? Yes, certainly, since they contribute to the improvement of techniques for individual identification and retrospective diagnosis (looking both at the pathophysiological condition of the subject and the causes and circumstances of death) through the application of anthropological methods of forensic science on osteo-archaeological evidence. Is this, then, a case of "biomedical research"? The texts defining this research, including in the international arena, are unambiguous: they concern "all research organized and practiced on human beings with a view to the development of biological and medical knowledge" (article L1121-1 of the Public Health Code of France).

The law of March 4, 2002 regulates medical confidentiality after death: it obliges the doctor to keep silent, except to research the causes of the disease or to improve the picture that could result from the disclosure of the medical file of the deceased. In addition, in the judicial framework of these postmortem studies, no consent is needed; does this then put the story and its understanding under the same imperative? It might be wise to place scientific knowledge and its research in the frame of humanism, which the Huriet-Sérusclat and then Jardé laws attempted to do. Henceforth, the law implicating people in a research project should involve all the human sciences, reaching far beyond the health sciences to include history, ethnology, and anthropology. But under what conditions?

Another question: can everything be published? Can one publish, in a widely distributed international journal, the photograph of the vulva of the mummy of a Spanish aristocrat, whose name and title are mentioned, who died over four centuries ago, who carried a tumor related to a vene-real disease? The caption notes that Maria of Aragon was wearing valuable clothing. Thus she had to be undressed for the study or . . . for the photo?

A doctor undertaking biomedical research on a patient is required to obtain the subject's consent when personal data or data allowing the possibility of identification are involved. If consent is impossible, some descendants may make themselves known, particularly if an image of the deceased and his dignity have not been respected. The cases of Ötzi and Tutankhamun, because of their cultural and chronological distance and the practice of "biomolecular Egyptology," can provoke questions of the same kind but, apparently, not with the same intensity. What sort of humanity are we speaking of? Indeed, let us not forget that what might be seen here as immodest (even voyeuristic) might not be so elsewhere; the sense of body and of its representations varies with different cultures, education, religions, and the chrono-cultural context.

Can time, therefore, be a discriminating element? Is there a period after which publications of this nature would carry no restrictions? Questioned on this subject, Dr. Irène Kahn (vice-president of the Conseil national de l'ordre des médecins [French Medical Board]) answered that the remains of subjects deceased long ago are similar to archives, and that consequently, it is the time restrictions placed on free access to health archives (medical records or hospital archives) that could be used by extrapolation—in other words, according to article L213-2 of the Heritage Code, 150 years after the death of the subject. But a reform currently under way could soon reduce this time to 120 years after the birth of the subject in question, or 25 years after his or her death.

How do such circumstances affect the respect for professional confidentiality? In practice, we would "violate" it only if it concerned our patient, but are these bodies, who have come from the past, who did not choose to be studied by us, really "patients" in the modern sense of the term? Or are they simply subjects of study, in the same way as an individual is who subjects him- or herself to a Phase III experiment[6] (indeed, is the investigating doctor or promoter facing a cohort of patients or simply facing subjects of investigation?). Rather, they are "deceased people," not people in the judicial sense, but in the sense of an entity without life, which is no longer a breathing subject, but who still deserves respect.

What does the Code of Ethics say? Article R4127-4 of the Public Health Code (in other words, the Code of Medical Ethics integrated within this more general code) states clearly:

> Professional confidentiality instituted in the interests of the patients is imposed on all doctors in the circumstances established by law. The confidentiality covers everything that the doctor has come to know in the practice of his profession, in other words, not only what has been confided to him, but also what he has seen, heard, or understood.

Does this apply to archaeological skeletons and mummies studied by doctors? In principle, no: the reference to "the interests of the patients" does not seem to be appropriate.

The fact remains that the motives of the authors of these publications are rather uncertain. . . . Are they seeking to generate awareness? Of what? To pique the curiosity of the reader (including through voyeurism)? It is not the legitimacy of medico-historical studies that is being questioned (even though one may have reservations regarding their intrusiveness into the intimacy of a family), but the spread of information without respect for the person and his or her privacy. This consideration can cause problems insofar as it questions the very meaning of biomedical research. All concerns that question, through ethics—more specifically, bioethics—the meaning of progress and innovation appear to be embarrassing.

Anonymization of any material before publication could be a minimum requirement (except when the point of the research happens to be the identification of an individual—like the head of Henri IV was recently).[7] The "thing" or injury that needs to be shown to demonstrate the case can be isolated from its context, as it is in the operating theatre. One could equally well present a histological section or a 3D reconstruction from a scanner rather than a photograph of genitals. Or simply cover the genitals of a mummy, as if it were any other patient, alive or dead.

In addition, could it not be a requirement that we publish only works in which the researcher himself, in the methodology, puts forward the arguments respecting the person being studied (a double responsibility, of the author and of the editor)? The editorial committee could refuse an article on this basis, stating the reason for its refusal.

Does the solution perhaps lie in a legal change to the status of the human body? Or in reflecting on the use of the word "person," including after death? The reason for asking this is that we need to establish (or develop) a code of ethics for the representation of knowledge, the conditions of scientific integrity and probity, and of practices in human sciences. Has the question already been asked? Is it not asked by the researchers themselves, when they offer suggestions to the law-makers that recognize the acceptance of these attitudes and behavior toward subjects who are sometimes several generations removed, toward deceased people? So that they should not simply be objects of research, but become human again,[8] part of the long line of humanity that continues to grow.

On the other hand, if we believe that science demands information about our ancestors that will be of benefit to everyone (requirements of culture, knowledge, the evolution of the person, etc.), we then find ourselves facing the need for research to be done on humans. Since, obviously, there can be no consent, one has to stand in a different epistemological place than ethics: that of moral obligation. This need can be elevated to the same status as justice, that is to say, the evidence of and the search for the demonstration of truth (for example with autopsies in a forensic context). In other words, to refer to a different vision of medical confidentiality, with the complete exemption from consent . . . which, in this context of the stakes of knowledge for society, does not preclude the preservation of modesty.

These thoughts also lead to relative moderation. To be human is to transmit through the filter of sensibility, necessity, elegance, case by case. To be scientific is to report on what is, by showing it when necessary, but without losing the dimension of respect owed to human remains, all of which participate in the future of humanity.

## Notes

1. Article co-authored with C. Huriet, Y. Coppens and C. Hervé, published in the *Revue de médecine légale*, 5, 2014, pp. 53–55.

2. Z. Hawass, Y. Z. Gad, S. Ismail *et al.*, "Ancestry and Pathology in King Tutankhamun's Family," Journal of the American Medical Association, 303/7, 2010, pp. 638–647.

3. G. Fornaciari, K. Zavaglia, L. Giusti *et al.*, "Human Papillomavirus in a 16th Century Mummy," *The Lancet*, 362, 2003, p. 1160.

4. W. F. Kean, S. Tocchio, M. Kean, K. D. Rainsford, "The Musculoskeletal Abnormalities of the Similaun Iceman ("Ötzi"): Clues to Chronic Pain and Possible Treatments," *Inflammopharmacol*, 21, 2013, pp. 11–20.

5. W.H.S. Jones (trans), *Hippocrates*, Volume 1, Loeb Classical Library 147, 1923, pp. 298–299.

6. Clinical trial carried out on patients comparing the efficiency of a new molecule with an old treatment and a placebo.

7. P. Charlier, *et al.*, "Multidisciplinary Medical Identification of a French King's Head (Henri IV)," *op. cit.*

8. P. Charlier, "Naming the Body (or the Bones): Human Remains, Anthropological/Medical Collections, Religious Beliefs, and Restitution," *Clinical Anatomy*, 27/3, 2014, pp. 291–295.

# Table 1. Vocabulary used for elementary lesions on dry bones

Based on P. Charon, "Méthodologie du diagnostic rétrospectif," in P. Charlier (ed.)
*Ostéo-archéologie et techniques médico-légales*, Paris, De Boccard, 2008, pp. 29–44.

| Macroscopic terms | |
|---|---|
| Erosion | Loss of cortical bone |
| Cavity | A resorptive depression |
| Perforation | Piercing or penetration of cortical bone |
| Osteolysis | Loss of substance through destruction of bone |
| Cortical fissure | A linear defect in cortical bone |
| Periostitis | A sub-periosteal deposit of newly formed bone on the cortical bone surface |
| Osteophytosis | Irregular bony growth found close to or on the articular surface of a bone |
| Exostosis | A projection of bony growth on the surface of a bone |
| Eburnation | Polishing of articular bone by bone-to-bone contact due to loss of cartilage; has the appearance of ivory |
| Osteopenia | Loss of trabecular bone with corresponding increase in the size of the medullary canal |
| Axial deformation | Modification of the axis of a bone by angulation, curving, or distortion |
| Deformation | Change in the shape of bone, dysplastic bone |
| Pseudoarthrosis | A false joint that forms between broken segments of a bone through continued movement |
| Ankylosis | Loss of joint movement through the fusion of two or more bones |
| Foreign bodies | Non-osseous bodies present in the bone tissue, which originate from the external environment |
| Blunted | Dull or rounded |
| Sharp | Fine or sharp margin |
| Regular | Uniform |
| Irregular | Non-uniform |

| | |
|---|---|
| Homogenous | Made of elements of the same sort |
| Heterogeneous | Made of elements of different sorts |
| Systemic | Organized according to an identifiable anatomical or anatamo-pathological system |
| Localized | Limited to a segment or part of a bone |
| Generalized | Spread across the whole bone |
| Articular | Located on the surface of a joint |
| Juxta-articular | Located next to a joint |
| Diaphyseal | Relating to the diaphysis of the bone |
| Metaphyseal | Relating to the metaphysis of the bone |
| Epiphyseal | Relating to the epiphysis of a bone |
| Compact bone | Bone having the structure of physiological bony cortical tissue |
| Cribiform bone | Compact bony tissue pierced by more or less numerous holes of various sizes |
| Cancellous or trabecular bone | Bone having the structure of spongy bone tissue |
| Porous bone | A bone with many holes (pores) in it, like trabecular bone |
| Nodular bone | Compact bone forming dense knobs of bone |
| Bone spicule | A slender projection of compact bone |
| **Radiology terms** | |
| Radiolucent | Reduction in the density of bone, which appears black on a radiograph |
| Lacuna, geode | A depressed lesion or depression in bone circumscribed by increased bone density |
| Trait or characteristic | An area of increased radio-opaque or radio-density of bone on a radiograph |
| Radio-dense | Sclerosis due to increased density of bone on a radiographic image, appears white on a radiograph |
| Diffuse | Spread broadly on a bone or among many bones |
| Disseminated | Spreading to parts that were not the original location of infection |
| Peripheral condensation | Sclerosis due to increased radio-density around a bony lesion |

| Medullary | Related to the medullary cavity or marrow canal of a bone |
|---|---|
| Endosteum | Related to the walls of the medullary cavity |
| Cortical | Related to the cortical bone |
| Sub-periosteal | On the surface of the cortical bone, forming beneath the periosteum |

## Table 2. Classification of traumatic cranial lesions

Based on G. Quatrehomme, V. Alunni-Perret, "Les lésions crâniennes tranchantes et contondantes en anthropologie médico-légale: étude préliminaire," *Journal de médecine légale droit médical*, 5/49, 2006, pp. 173–189.

| Lesions | | | Mechanisms |
|---|---|---|---|
| Bruised bone | | | Blunt force trauma, without great force |
| Break in bone surface | Erosion | | Low energy blunt force / Perpendicular or oblique blow / Tangential blow, more or less violent |
| | Penetration | Shape of the weapon responsible (regular edges, no radiating fractures) | Cutting or piercing |
| | Perforation | Rough shape (irregular edges, associated radiating fractures) | Blunt force |
| | Avulsion | (irregular edges, associated fractures, frequent plastic deformation) | |
| Radiating | (radial or concentric fractures, isolated or accompanying a loss of bone continuity) | | |
| Depressed | (often with radiating and concentric fractures, irregular edges, plastic deformation of bones, diastatic fractures and comminution) | | |

# SUGGESTED READING

Andrieux P., Hadjouis D., Dambricourt-Malassé A., *L'Identité humaine en question. Nouvelles problématiques et nouvelles technologies en paléontologie humaine et en paléo-anthropologie biologique*, Paris, Art'com, 2000.

Ariès P., *Essais sur l'histoire de la mort en Occident du Moyen Âge à nos jours*, Paris, Éd. du Seuil, 1975.

Beaumont E., *Vanikoro. Journal d'un médecin légiste sur "l'île du Malheur" où périt Lapérouse*, Tahiti, Au vent des îles, 2004.

Berriot-Salvadore E. (ed.), *Ambroise Paré, une vive mémoire*, Paris, De Boccard, 2012.

Boëtsch G., Hervé C., Rozenberg J.-J., *Corps normalisé, corps stigmatisé, corps radicalisé*, Bruxelles, De Boeck, 2007.

Brothwell D. R., *Digging up Bones: The Excavation, Treatment and Study of Human Skeletal Remains*, London, British Museum, 1963.

Canci A., Minozzi S., *Archeologia dei resti umani*, Rome, Carocci, 2005.

Castex D., Cartron I. (eds), *Epidémies et crises de mortalité du passé*, Bordeaux, Ausonius, 2007.

Charlier P. (ed.), *Ostéo-archéologie et techniques médico-légales*, Paris, De Boccard, 2008.

Collard F., Samama E. (eds), *Handicaps et sociétés dans l'histoire. L'estropié, l'aveugle et le paralytique de l'Antiquité aux Temps modernes*, Paris, L'Harmattan, 2010.

Crubézy E., Duchesne S., Arlaud C. (eds), *La Mort, les Morts et la Ville (Montpellier, X–XVIᵉ siècle)*, Paris, Errance, 2006.

Delabarde T., Ludes B. (ed.), *Manuel pratique d'anthropologie médico-légale*, Paris, ESKA, 2014.

Durigon M., Guénanten M., *Pratique de la thanatopraxie*, Paris, Masson, 2009.

Erlande-Brandenbourg A., *Le roi est mort. Étude sur les funérailles, les sépultures et les tombeaux des rois de France jusqu'à la fin du XIIIᵉ siècle*, Paris, Arts et métiers graphiques, 1975.

Fisher B.A.J., Svensson A., Wendel O., *Techniques of Crime Scene Investigation*, New York, Elsevier, 1987.

Gourevitch D., *Le Triangle hippocratique dans le monde gréco-romain. Le malade, sa maladie et son médecin*, Paris, De Boccard, 1984.

Guilaine J., Zammit J., *Le Sentier de la guerre. Visages de la violence préhistorique*, Paris, Éd. du Seuil, 2001.

Guy H., Jeanjean A., Richier A. (eds), *Le Cadavre en procès*, Marseille, Techniques et cultures, 2013.

King H., Dasen V., *La Médecine dans l'Antiquité grecque et romaine*, Lausanne, BHMS, 2008.

Le Breton D., *La Chair à vif. Usages médicaux et mondains du corps humain*, Paris, Métailié, 1993.

Lopez G, Tzitzis S (eds), *Dictionnaire des sciences criminelles*, Paris, Dalloz, 2004.

Ménenteau S., *L'Autopsie judiciaire. Histoire d'une pratique ordinaire au XIX^e siècle*, Rennes, PUR, 2013.

Perez S., *La Mort des rois*, Grenoble, Jérôme Millon, 2006.

Schnitzler B, Le Minor J.-M., Ludes B., Boës E. (eds), *Histoire(s) de squelettes. Archéologie, médecine et anthropologie en Alsace*, Strasbourg, Musées de Strasbourg, 2005.

Thiel M.-J. (ed.), *Les Rites autour du mourir*, Strasbourg, Presses universitaires de Strasbourg, 2008.

Thomas L. V., *Rites de mort, pour la paix des vivants*, Paris, Fayard, 1985.

Vons J. (ed.), *Pratique et pensée médicales à la Renaissance*, Paris, De Boccard, 2009.

Wells C., *Bones, Bodies and Disease*, New York, Praeger, 1964.

# ACKNOWLEDGMENTS

None of the studies mentioned above could have been undertaken without a real and constructive interdisciplinarity. So it is that the following researchers worked on these patients from the past, for which we thank them very warmly: I. Abadie, A. Alduc-Le Bagousse, J.-P. Babelon, A. Baralis, R. Bianucci, M. Billard, J. Blondiaux, R. Boano, S. Bohic, F. Bouchet, C. Brombacher, L. Brun, C. Buquet-Marion, P.-F. Campos, R. Carlier, P. Catalano, S. Cavard, P.-F. Chaillot, G. Cheylan, G. Costea, M. Cotte, A. Cotten, S. Delacourte, S. Descamps, L. Devisme, S. Digiannantonio, C. Dorion-Peyronnet, E. de Dreuzy, P. Dubrisay, R. Durand, J.-M. Duriez, M. Durigon, A. Eb, L. Eisenberg, S. El-Balkhi, A. Embs, A. Etcheberry, D. Favier, O. Ferrant, D. Fompeydie, P. Froesch, A. Froment, S. Gabet, B. Galland, P. Georges, T. Gilbert, Y. Glon, M. Goubard, D. Gourevitch, R. Grilletto, S. Harter-Lalheugue, C. Hervé, A. Hurel, I. Huynh-Charlier, G.-F. Jeannel, H. Jouin-Spriet, C. Keyser, S. Khung-Savatovsky, C. Lalueza-Fox, E. Lancelot, L. Laquay, A.-M. Lazar, M. Le Bailly, J.-L. Lemaître, Y. Lemoine, C. Le Roy, L. Lo Gerfo, Y. Loublier, B. Ludes, V. Lungu, F. Masson, P. de Mazancourt, V. Mazel, A. Moirin, R. Montagut, D. Morillon, C. Moulherat, O. Munoz, Y. Neuzillet, F. Pannier, W. Pantano, M. Patou-Mathis, J. Perot, S.-M. Popescu, J. Poupon, C. Prêtre, F. Reynaud, P. Richardin, M. Rippa Bonati, L. Robbiola, H. Rossinot, N. Rouquet, A. Samzun, J.-F. Saliège, A. L. Schällin, B. Sendid, P. Sorel, A. I. Sundström, J. Susini, S. Thiébault, P. L. Thillaud, X. Trufaut, C. Tsigonaki, Y. Ubelmann, A.-M. Verhille, J.-N. Vignal, F. Wallet, R. Weil, and E. Willerslev.

David Alliot wishes to thank Philippe Charlier for his trust and availability; Mr. Joël Poupon, as one should, on earth and in heaven; Mr. Patrick Rainsard, who makes us laugh; Mr. Xavier de Bartillat from the éditions Tallandier; as well as Ms. Dominique Missika, for her constant and friendly concern.

The authors wish to express their gratitude to Mr. Philippe Druillet, their perpetual and permanent source of inspiration, who will be a fabulous archaeological case in a few centuries.

PHILIPPE CHARLIER, MD PhD LittD (forensics, anthropology, ethics), is head of the section of medical and forensic anthropology at the University of Versailles at St. Quentin. He is a specialist in rituals related to diseases and death and has been christened by the press "the Indiana Jones of the graveyards." He is the author of *Zombies: An Anthropological Investigation of the Living Dead.*

DAVID ALLIOT, a trainer at the National Institute of Training of the Librairie (INFL, France), is passionate about the forms of language and books, and works as an independent publisher of different French publishing houses, specializing in the writer Louis-Ferdinand Céline and the Martinique poet Aimé Césaire.

ISABELLE RUBEN is a freelance archaeologist with over forty years' experience. Having graduated from the University of London with a degree in archaeology, she has worked in contract archaeology across the United States and currently lives and works in Jordan, participating in or managing innumerable archaeological projects throughout the Middle East. Being freelance allows for a wide range of work opportunities and, apart from archaeology, these have included writing, editing, translating, book layout, tour guiding, and tour development. With particular interest in the natural world, Isabelle has written and produced a book field guide to the plants and animals of the Petra area in Jordan. Other books that she has edited and produced include a book on the Petra Siq, one on the dolmens of Jordan, and one on the history of the Jordan InterContinental Hotel.